NAVIGATING
THE MEDICAL MAZE

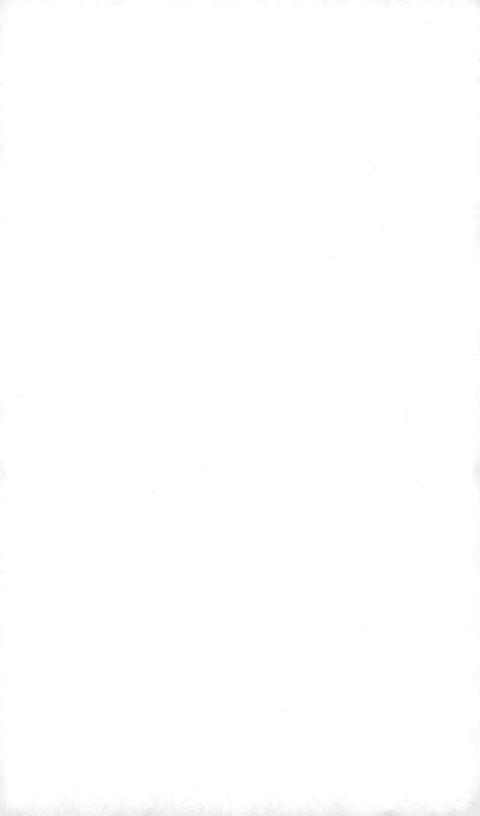

NAVIGATING
THE MEDICAL MAZE

A PRACTICAL GUIDE

STEVEN L. BROWN

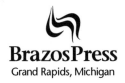

Brazos Press
Grand Rapids, Michigan

Published by Brazos Press
a division of Baker Publishing Group
P.O. Box 6287, Grand Rapids, MI 49516-6287
www.brazospress.com

Printed in the United States of America

This book gives general information about medical issues to make you a more informed healthcare consumer. It does not provide individualized advice for particular health problems. We have endeavored to ensure that it is accurate at the time of publication. However, since medical knowledge is continually growing and changing, some information in this book may no longer be current at the time you read it. Because of these limitations, this book cannot take the place of a personal evaluation by a healthcare professional.

Library of Congress Cataloging-in-Publication Data
Brown, Steven L., 1959–
    Navigating the medical maze : a practical guide / Steven L. Brown.
        p. cm.
    Includes bibliographical references.
    ISBN 10: 1-58743-207-2 (pbk.)
    ISBN 978-1-58743-207-1 (pbk.)
    1. Medical care—United States. 2. Physicians. 3. Alternative medicine.
4. Health. I. Title.
RA776.B795 2007
610—dc22   2007013279

Contents

Acknowledgments   7

1. Thrown into the Medical Maze   9

PART 1:

THE DOCTOR

2. Steering Clear of Bad Doctors   21
3. How to Recognize the Best Doctors   31
4. Support Your Local Doctor   55

PART 2:

THE PRINCIPLES

5. How Do We Know If a Treatment Works?   71
6. Does Bias Affect Everyone, Even My Doctors
   and Me?   95
7. Avoiding the Traps That Bias Sets for
   You   107

PART 3:

ALTERNATIVE MEDICINE

8. Is Alternative Medicine Better Than
   Conventional Medicine?   137

9. Dying of Natural Causes: Alternative
   Medicines Aren't Dangerous, Are They?   151
10. How Can I Tell If the Evidence Is Any
    Good?   171
11. What about Other Claims Made by Some
    Alternative Practitioners?   197

PART 4:

THE PATIENT

12. How Can I Deal with My Illness?   217
13. Frequently Asked Questions   235
14. How Can I Live a Healthy Life?   249

Acknowledgments

The suffering I have seen caused by bad medical advice motivated me to write this book. I dedicate it to the families whose pain I have seen. I hope its contents will prevent suffering in the lives of others.

Many friends have helped me through this long process, with words of encouragement, suggestions about parts of the manuscript, and questions about progress. I especially thank Preston and Susan Abbott, James and Cindy Bobo, David and Susan Brown, David and Cindy DeShan, Tim and Terri Dunn, Tim and Lisa Frosch, Mark and Colleen McLane, Clay and Christa Midkiff, Mike Miller, Randy and Amy Sims, and Peggy Waisanen. Providentially, Lee and Ellen Vaughn and Denny Boultinghouse were there to help me immeasurably just when I needed them. Andy Krafsur and Greg Frost provided important direction with business issues. Dr. Paul Reisser thoroughly reviewed the entire manuscript and provided numerous helpful suggestions. I deeply appreciate his help, given at a time when he had many other responsibilities.

I am most grateful for the professionals at Brazos Press. Rodney Clapp's vision for the book and his editorial expertise were invaluable. I also especially thank Rebecca Cooper and B.J. Heyboer.

Dina McCormick, the nurse who is my right hand in the office, has been a great help by providing encouragement, ideas, and suggestions. She is the principle educator in my practice. Her knowledge of what the average person understands was most helpful in developing this book.

Most importantly, I thank my family for their understanding and patience. My wife, Tamarah, has been the perfect helpmeet. She served as my initial reader and editor. Without her expertise and honest criticism, this book would not exist. I cannot express how deeply I appreciate her support for me and her care for our family during this process.

1

✚

Thrown into the Medical Maze

"CODE BLUE! ROOM 7! EMERGENCY ROOM!"

The hospital public-address system crackled overhead. Julie's shiny blond hair cascaded over the end of the stretcher where the respiratory therapist stood, his left hand holding the mask over her face and his right hand squeezing the Ambu-bag every three seconds to deliver pure oxygen to her lungs. The orderly was leaning over her pale, lifeless body, the heel of his palm over her breastbone, pressing down once each second to circulate her blood. Her heart had stopped only a few seconds before and was now fibrillating, quivering like a sack of worms, instead of pumping as it had for the past thirty-eight years. A nurse placed an adhesive-backed electrode the size of an open hand on her chest, just to the right of the sternum, and another in her armpit, just beside her left breast. The air of the hospital felt even colder than usual as we all looked down at Julie.

"Charge to 200," I said, as the nurse pressed the appropriate button.

"All clear!"

After confirming that no one was touching her body or the stretcher, I pushed the two red buttons simultaneously, and the defibrillator shocked her heart. We all looked up at the monitor. Everyone began to breathe again as the monitor came to life, beeping regularly as her heart returned to a normal rhythm.

"Let's get a blood pressure." The nurse was already leaning over Julie's arm with a stethoscope in her ears.

"85/50," she replied.

"Let's *move!*" I ordered. The respiratory therapist secured the oxygen canister beneath the stretcher as the nurse hooked the monitoring electrodes to the portable unit.

As we rushed down the hall to the cardiac catheterization laboratory, I thought back over the story that Julie had told me in the half-hour before her heart stopped. Her gynecologist told her a year ago that her cholesterol was high. She tried to control it with diet and exercise; although she continued to smoke, she actually embarked on a jogging program. It had had little effect, but Julie had no warning that she might be developing a heart problem.

Yesterday at around 3:30 p.m., she had felt a tight sensation in her chest. She thought it might be indigestion, although she had not had any problems with indigestion before. She considered calling her doctor but did not know what she would do with her two children, aged six and eight, if she had to go to his office. This morning, Julie had been increasingly short of breath and finally almost passed out when she got up from a chair. She got a neighbor to bring her to the emergency room. When she arrived at about 9:30 a.m., an EKG showed that she was having a massive heart attack, and the emergency-room doctor had called me immediately.

A heart attack occurs because a clot forms in one of the arteries to the heart, cutting off the blood supply. The doctor's primary objective is to get the artery open as quickly as possible. If the artery is opened less than thirty minutes after the onset of symptoms, there is often no damage at all. However, as time goes by, more and more heart muscle dies. Most of the damage is done within twelve hours, and the heart continues to deteriorate up to twenty-four hours after symptom onset. Unfortunately in Julie's case, after eighteen hours a lot of damage had already been done. Her blood pressure was low now because her heart had grown quite weak. This condition is called cardiogenic shock, and it carries a very high risk of death. In addition, because of the weakening of the heart, fluid had built up in her lungs to the point that she required 100 percent oxygen to stay alive. I had told her husband that she was at high risk for dying, no matter what we did.

After we moved Julie from the stretcher onto the x-ray table, an anesthesiologist placed a tube through her throat into her lungs to ensure adequate oxygen delivery from the breathing machine. At the same time, the cardiac catheterization laboratory nurses and x-ray technicians applied additional EKG electrodes and prepared her for the sterile procedure. When everything was ready, I threaded catheters up to the heart via the artery in her right leg. We found what we expected: the artery going down the front of the heart was totally blocked.

Carefully, I pushed a soft-tipped wire across the blockage, opening a tiny channel for blood to flow. Her heart stopped once again, and again restarted beating after a single shock. Using a specially designed catheter, we sucked a clot out of the blocked artery. I then carefully placed a tiny metal tubular mesh, called a stent, precisely where the artery was blocked. I inflated a balloon within the stent to embed it in the artery. Although the x-ray screen showed that the artery was now wide open, a lot of damage had been done to Julie's heart while the artery was closed.

She began to awaken later that night. Although she could not speak because the tube going into her lungs went through her voice box, her husband was able to tell her what had happened. The next day, blood tests showed that her liver had been damaged by the shock she had undergone, but her kidneys, fortunately, were intact. Her lungs were still so full of fluid that she continued to need the breathing machine.

Over the next few days, I helped Julie get rid of the excess fluid in her lungs using medications. Finally, four days after she was admitted, she was able to breathe on her own. By this time her liver had also recovered. With physical therapy, she began to regain her strength. She received a lot of education about heart disease, cholesterol, and smoking cessation.

Doctors have studied heart attacks more extensively than most health problems. In part, this is because heart attacks kill so many people. Perhaps the fact that they occur frequently in affluent middle-aged men also plays a role in the allocation of those research dollars. Congestive heart failure—accumulation of fluid in the body due weakening of the heart muscle—has been studied extensively for the same reasons.

Because of these studies, we know that people like Julie are likely to live longer and recover more fully if they are given a combination of medications at certain doses. During her two weeks in the hospital, I initiated these medications gradually and adjusted the doses slowly, so that by the time of discharge, we had made a good start on ensuring her health.

Now it is a month later. Julie is seated in my office, her cheeks pink and her face smiling. Nonetheless, there is worry in her eyes. Her husband is with her, and his face is also fearful. Her EKG shows extensive damage to her heart from her heart attack. As I pull her blue gown aside to listen to her heart, I can tell that the heart muscle is severely weakened. Still, she is getting stronger and feels better daily.

Thinking that their anxiety is about her future, I begin to discuss her prognosis. Her risk of death in the next year is still significant, but she has survived the time of highest risk, and the fact that she has done well so far is encouraging. Looking a little embarrassed, Julie explains that this is not why she is anxious today.

"Dr. Brown," she begins, "my friends tell me that medicines are dangerous, but that if I'll just take these natural supplements I bought at the health food store, I will get well."

Her husband hoists a large paper sack containing no fewer than twenty bottles. There is desperation in their voices. They hope that these pills recommended by their friends will be like a Tree of Life, bringing immortality without any risk. Although they still trust me enough to ask my opinion, they are now afraid of the medications that I have prescribed to keep Julie alive.

This scenario plays out many times a day in my office and in the offices of doctors all over the world. It's quite understandable. Any illness brings our frailty and mortality up to the surface of our consciousness. We long to be given treatments that will restore our health. More than that, we want to avoid doing anything that might make us even worse. Competing claims assault us in print, in the mail, and on television. On the one hand, there are claims that doctors or drug companies are evil and dishonest. On the other hand, news reports describe triumphs of modern medicine in curing disease and improving quality and quantity of life. On the one hand, we hear about the horribleness of disease. On the other hand, the Internet is filled with claims that we can have health "without surgery or drugs." Whom can we trust? Whom do we believe? How can we decide what to do? How can so many seemingly intelligent, caring people reach such different conclusions?

"Julie, let's look at some broader issues. With your heart attack you have entered a new continent—the continent of health care. You need to learn how to travel safely through it. It is a dark continent: no one travels here unless they have to, because there is at least some danger and uncertainty in every city, town, and village. It actually feels like a maze, since you will often feel hemmed in and not know which way to turn. But now that you have a health problem, you have no choice but to travel here. With the right education, your journey can be as safe as possible and can even be pleasant. But you must stay alert and know how to choose the right path."

Perhaps you or someone you love is facing a new health problem. You have done what you could to stay healthy, but now the doctor says that you have high blood pressure, or high cholesterol, or cancer, or heart failure. Perhaps your mother or father is facing Alzheimer's disease and looks to you for direction. Now the continent you had avoided stretches before you—the dark continent of health care. You have to go there to get what you need, but you do not understand the customs and dangers of this strange land. You do not want just to have someone tell you what to do, although there are plenty of voices clamoring to do just that. You want to understand the issues for yourself and be equipped to make your own decisions. The whole situation makes your heart stop, and you need help to get it going again.

This book will give you the equipment you need to answer these questions for yourself, your family, and your loved ones. I spend hours each week talking to people like you about health issues. I have seen bad health decisions cause damage, death, and devastation. I have seen excessive medical care kill people. I have seen inadequate medical care kill people. To make wise health decisions, you *need* to understand the issues involved.

In the first part of the book, I will discuss the strengths and weaknesses of modern medicine, with a particular focus on medical doctors. Your doctor is, unavoidably, your personal guide on this trip. Like tour guides for any expedition, some are good, and some are bad. A few are more interested in making money than in helping you. Many are mediocre. A few are outstanding. As a doctor myself, I have seen the good, the bad, and the ugly. I will help you understand our training and how we look at things, so that you will know how to get the best medical care for your family. I will help you find an excellent doctor and build a strong relationship with him or her.

In part 2, I discuss the principles that allowed great progress in medicine in the past century. The purpose of this part of the book is to give you the navigational tools that you need. This section includes a lot of discussion of *bias*, the lack of objectivity that afflicts all of us. If you want to get along in the strange land of health care, you need to understand the darker part of the culture, and this section will give you that understanding. When you finish this part of the book, you will understand how to read a map and use a compass.

In part 3, we will join Julie on her pilgrimage to understand the issues surrounding what has been called complementary and alternative medicine. You may be surprised to learn that there are risks associated with these treatments. I will give you the tools you need to evaluate the options in this confusing part of the continent.

Finally, in part 4, I turn away from looking at the health-care system and turn my attention to our experience as patients. The "traveling tips" in this section of the book will help make your travel experience a more pleasant one. We will review some of the emotional aspects of dealing with illness. I will tie together principles from the rest of the book by answering some FAQs (frequently asked questions). I will bring the issues of health into perspective with a few broad principles and some thoughts about how health issues fit into the rest of life. I hope that this section will serve as a great encouragement if you are facing new health problems, and that it will get you to the oases in the vast deserts of this continent.

Throughout the book, you will read stories about people just like yourself. Because of confidentiality, unless I am citing a report published elsewhere, all the individuals I discuss are fictitious. I wouldn't want to read my own medical history in a book, so if one of these fictitious patients even *reminded* me of someone, I did all I could to make sure that the stories did not match real cases. But while the patients are imaginary, the problems they face are all too common and all too real.

My perspective on health issues is shaped by my Christian view of the world. I will explain a Christian worldview of health care and contrast it to other philosophies. These parts of the text will be separated into shaded boxes. If you share a Christian perspective, these sections will be an additional inspiration to you. If you don't, I hope that you find it illuminating to realize that our philosophical views of the world have such concrete implications.

After you read this book, you will have an insider's view of some of the critical issues in twenty-first-century health care. More often than you imagine now, the issues are the same as issues in the rest of society, played out on the field of health care. Most important, however, you will understand how to protect your own health and how to navigate through the maze of conflicting advice to arrive at the best choices for you and your family.

PART **1**

✚

THE
DOCTOR

2

✚

Steering Clear
of Bad Doctors

When a doctor goes wrong, he is the first of criminals. He has nerve and he has knowledge.

Sherlock Holmes in
"The Adventure of the Speckled Band"

"Julie, the person, other than yourself, whom you rely on the most in this journey of health care is the doctor. Your doctor is like a personal guide for the trip. And the trip is more like a hiking adventure up a mountain or through a rain forest than like a trip to a resort."

"Dr. Brown, you can say that again."

"Choosing the right guide for the trip is your most important decision. Have you heard any stories about doctors who were dishonest?"

"I sure have. I have heard of doctors doing unnecessary surgery or doing sloppy work and hurting people."

"Julie, that is a real problem. Let me show you just how bad it really is."

A Redding Surgery Mill

John Corapi has an inspiring story. He was very successful in real estate and then fell into drug use. Ultimately, after hitting bottom, he returned to the church, attended seminary, and became a priest. His ministry now involves traveling all over the world as a speaker.[1]

At a friend's suggestion, Corapi went to see Dr. Chae Hyun Moon, a cardiologist in Redding, California, where Corapi resides. Dr. Moon did a stress test and subsequently recommended an angiogram. After the procedure, while Corapi was still on the table, Moon leaned over and told him that he needed triple bypass surgery. Although he recommended that the surgery be done immediately, Corapi asked if it could be delayed long enough to allow him to fly to Norfolk, Virginia, to speak to an audience of Pentagon officials, and Moon agreed.[2]

Corapi spoke with a friend in Las Vegas whose girlfriend was a nurse in a critical care unit there. His friend offered to let Corapi stay with him after the surgery so he would have help and company during recuperation. Therefore, Corapi opted to have his surgery in Las Vegas instead.

When the doctors in Las Vegas reviewed his records, however, they told him that his heart was normal and that there was no need for surgery. Still worried, Corapi obtained a total of five doctors' opinions. All agreed that he needed no surgery.[3]

Corapi arranged a meeting with Redding Medical Center CEO Hal Chilton to raise concerns that Moon was encouraging patients to have unnecessary surgery. Instead of initiating an investigation, Chilton claimed that the Nevada doctors must have been mistaken, and he encouraged Corapi to proceed with surgery at his hospital. This was despite the fact that, as it turned out, several years before others had told Chilton about Moon's propensity to recommend unneeded surgery.[4]

Father Corapi went to the FBI, which initiated an investigation. Ultimately, the FBI alleged in an affidavit that as many as half of the procedures done by Dr. Moon and the surgeon to whom he referred, Dr. Fidel Realyvasquez, were not appropriate and that a quarter were done on patients with no heart problems. Tenet Healthcare, which owns the hospital involved, settled with the government for $54 million,and later settled civil lawsuits resulting from these revelations for $395 million.[5]

Do you think that being rich or famous is any protection from this type of dishonesty? Among the victims of this pair was country music star Merle Haggard.[6] How can any layperson know that she or he is being lied to by a doctor? In the worst-case scenario, a doctor is like a commission salesman whose customer has to buy whatever he recommends. The potential for abuse is staggering.

It Happens in Your Town, Too

Unfortunately, this problem is not limited to Redding, California. In my practice, I have seen a disturbing number of patients who have undergone unnecessary surgery. Sometimes the scam is quite complex.

Cindy was a single mother of two children, trying her best to make ends meet and raise her children well. She was in her early twenties and worked as a teacher's aide. Her job provided no health insurance. She went to see a

A Christian Perspective

Should dishonesty among physicians surprise us? From a Christian perspective, the answer is no. Your doctor is *fallen*, like Adam and Eve in the Garden of Eden. Just like all people, your doctor has a tendency toward sin. The prophet Isaiah tells us, "All of us like sheep have gone astray; each of us has turned to his own way" (Isa. 53:6). Even David, who was righteous early and late in his life, went through a period of evil, during which he was guilty of both adultery and murder.[7]

doctor because she had an upper respiratory infection. He treated her cold but also claimed that he heard something wrong with her heart; he recommended that she come back in for an EKG, which is a recording of the heart's electrical activity.

The day after the test, she received a telephone call from the doctor. He told her to come to his office right away, because he had terrible news for her.

Terrified, she drove to his office. After she sat down, he told her that she had a condition called "PVCs." She would never be able to work again. He would help her get on disability.

She discussed the situation with her mother, who knew that this doctor had a bad reputation. Cindy looked up PVCs in a medical book and learned that for the most part they are benign. Finally, at her mother's insistence, she came to see me for a second opinion.

PVCs, or premature ventricular contractions, are simply extra heartbeats. They can be a sign of an underlying heart problem, but in and of themselves, they are neither dangerous nor disabling. After a careful evaluation, I was able to determine that Cindy's heart was completely normal. And when I finally received a copy of the EKG in question, it turned out that it was completely normal: *she did not even have PVCs*. Unfortunately, because she had gone through the psychological process of accepting that she had a life-threatening problem, it was now hard for Cindy to believe that she was healthy.

Why would the doctor do this to her? His actions could have destroyed her life and damaged the lives of her children. As it turned out, this was his standard operating procedure. A patient with no insurance represented a very limited source of revenue. However, once he got the patient on disability, he could milk Medicare for large amounts of money, doing tests that she did not need for conditions that she did not have.

Fortunately, most doctors are honest, hardworking, responsible, and caring people who do their best to care for their patients and make great sacrifices to do so. But when a doctor is dishonest, the average patient has little defense. The same is true when the doctor is incompetent, lazy, ignorant, or irresponsible. Even more subtle is the problem of conflict of interest, where a doctor is convinced that her actions are reasonable but cannot see clearly due to her vested interest in the decision.

As in all areas of life, there are plenty of people who *are* honest. Some are honest for selfish reasons, believing that they will come out ahead in the end. Others are honest on principle. Some tell the truth because they fear the consequences of being caught in a lie. Yet all of us are capable of being honest or dishonest, good or evil. Recognizing this, we should not be paralyzed by fear, but we should maintain a healthy wariness in dealing with anyone.

The next chapter will discuss the training of physicians and how it builds into young doctors the values of honesty and self-sacrifice. This training reduces the amount of dishonesty that would otherwise be likely. The selection process for physicians also tends to favor those who have demonstrated commitment to selfless activities. As a result, fortunately, most doctors do conduct themselves honorably and are as horrified as you and I about acts of abuse such as those discussed above. When we see evidence of dishonesty, however, we must take it seriously.

Protecting Yourself

What can you do to protect yourself from dishonest doctors? The first step is prevention, by picking the best, most honest, most careful, most thorough doctor you can find. I will discuss this more in the next chapter.

However, sometimes you may find yourself in a situation where you are being abused and do not know it. What are some clues? How can you protect yourself?

1. *Take any hints about dishonesty very seriously.* I have seen a number of patients whose doctors have been sent to prison. I have heard some of these patients make statements like these:

> "He may have lied to other people, but I am sure that he was honest with *me*."
> "He was a good doctor; he was just a bad businessman."
> "He saved my life on several occasions."

All these statements reflect a frightening naiveté. We all want desperately to believe that our doctor is perfect, caring, honest, and meticulous, so we tend to discount indications to the contrary. However, we need to look objectively at any information that suggests a problem. Otherwise, we will misinterpret evidence of dishonesty as evidence of thoroughness. One patient whose doctor was ultimately sentenced to prison asserted stoutly, "This fine doctor has done seventeen surgical procedures on me within the past two years." Now I have not reviewed this patient's medical records, but to have one procedure done in two years is reasonable. To have three is sometimes appropriate. For a doctor to perform seventeen procedures on one patient in two years is almost always criminal.

2. *Do some of your own research.* Unfortunately, the Internet is a bit like a bathroom wall: anyone with a few minutes of privacy can write whatever he or she wants. Even university websites sometimes contain thinly veiled advertisements for treatments that are not proven but are offered at the facility sponsoring the site. However, the Internet is a vast and easily accessible resource for information, and university sites are safer than the many sites that offer easy cures for your condition.

When you receive a new diagnosis, be sure you have the exact name and spelling, and read about it on university websites or on sites that your doctor recommends. After you have read about the condition, discuss with your doctor the information you have obtained, and see what she says. While most doctors are frustrated with the amount of false information that we have to dismiss, we do want our patients to have plenty of accurate information, and we want to help clarify what they have read. In Cindy's case, doing some research delivered her and her children from a life of poverty.

3. *Do not hesitate to get a second opinion in a nonemergency situation.* An honest doctor will welcome the opportunity to help you get a second opinion for a nonemergency procedure. We would rather get your questions answered before you have an operation or a risky treatment than to have you suffer a complication from a treatment that you were not convinced you needed in the first place. I am not saying that everyone should always get a second

opinion; I am saying that if you are not comfortable with a recommendation and the procedure is elective, then you should consider it. It was a second opinion that saved Father Corapi from unnecessary heart surgery. In his case, assurances from several other doctors were almost thwarted by the original doctor's claim that his condition required this surgery as an emergency procedure.

In an emergency situation, a second opinion is not always possible. However, you usually know if you are in an emergency: you came to the hospital because you were having serious symptoms. If you come to the hospital with chest pain, for example, you may be having a heart attack, so the delay of even a few minutes would likely be harmful. If you come to the hospital with abdominal pain and the doctor is worried about appendicitis, it may not be appropriate to wait for a second opinion. In Corapi's case, however, the statement that surgery was an emergency requirement was hard to swallow, since Corapi had no cardiac symptoms. Further, his doctor backed down when Corapi asked for a delay.

4. *Be suspicious when you undergo multiple expensive tests every time you go to the doctor's office, even when you have no symptoms. Be equally suspicious when you go to the doctor's office with the same problem multiple times and no tests are done.* Stan Smith went to a doctor in a nearby city, often several times a year, and each time the doctor ordered an EKG and a twenty-four-hour heart monitor. That doctor was later sent to prison on drug charges. If every time you took your car to the shop you walked out with a bill for five hundred dollars, you would find another mechanic. When your doctor orders a test, ask why it is necessary. The doctor should be happy to explain.

On the other hand, if your doctor is lazy, he might not order any tests at all. Now, many problems can be diagnosed simply by listening to your story and examining you. However, if the doctor treats you but you don't get any better, you probably need more tests or an appointment with a doctor who specializes in your problem. For example, if I see a patient with chest discomfort that I believe is due to a stomach problem, I may treat her with a potent antiacid medication. If she returns to see me three weeks later and the pain is no better, I need to reexamine my diagnosis. That may mean doing a stress test to look for a heart problem, sending her to a stomach specialist, or sending her to a pain specialist, depending on the details of her symptoms.

5. *Rely on the advice of trusted medical advisers.* Before you find yourself in the situation of not knowing whether to trust your doctor, you need to establish yourself with a primary care doctor whom you can trust. How to establish such a relationship is discussed in the next chapter. That individual can then serve as your advocate and can advise you on choosing a specialist when one is needed.

Conclusion

This chapter has discussed some of the worst abuses of trust that can occur. When we go to a physician, we are entrusting our life to that person, trusting his or her stated commitment to our welfare. A doctor who hurts people for profit violates that sacred trust. Fortunately, this level of evil is rare in medicine. Unfortunately, however, mediocrity is all too common.

How can you tell the difference between excellence and mediocrity? We'll discuss that toward the end of the next chapter. But first, I want to introduce you to the world of medicine through the eyes of the physician.

Notes

1. Kelly St. John and Mark Martin, "Heart Patient's Many Lives: Redding Whistle-Blower Went from Riches to Rags to Robes," *San Francisco Chronicle*, November 10, 2002, A-1, www.sfgate.com/cgi-bin/article.cgi?f=/c/a/2002/11/10/MN67216.DTL&hw=john+corapi&sn=001&sc=1000 (accessed June 17, 2006).

2. Ibid.; Ronald D. White, "Priest's Heart 'Trauma' Triggers Tenet Probe," *Los Angeles Times*, November 5, 2002, www.csudh.edu/dear habermas/medfraudbk01.htm (accessed June 17, 2006).

3. Ibid.

4. St. John and Martin, "Heart Patient's Many Lives."

5. Kim Dixon, "Tenet Settles Heart Surgery Lawsuits for $395 Million," December 21, 2004, www.vascularweb.org/_CONTRIBUTION_PAGES/Medical_News_Reuters/Tenet_Settles_Heart_Surgery_Lawsuits.html (accessed September 25, 2005).

6. "Tenet Suit Alleges Unneeded Heart Surgery," August 17, 2003, www.yourlawyer.com/articles/read/6462 (accessed June 17, 2006).

7. The story is told in 2 Samuel 11–12.

3

✚

How to Recognize
the Best Doctors

"Dr. Brown," Julie continued, "I actually asked around about you while I was in the hospital and since I got out. You have a good reputation, and I believe that you have my best interests at heart. Is that true of most doctors?"

"Julie, most doctors are honest and will work hard for you. Part of the reason for that is the training that we go through."

Basic Training

It is at least 100 degrees and dripping-with-sweat humid. The movie set looks exactly like the Marine Corps Recruit Depot on Parris Island, South Carolina. The young actors stand on the steaming asphalt in various caricatures of "attention" as the actor playing the drill instructor eye-balls each one from head to toe. Even though I am in an air-conditioned theater, the images so completely communication the combination of heat, tension, and fear that I almost taste the sweat on my own face.

As usual in this type of film, the characters represent a cross-section of American society. The proud high school athlete is standing straight up with his smirk and sunglasses. The frightened fat guy throws his shoulders back as far as they will go. The gum-chewing racist white guy is slouching next to the serious, honorable black man who will become the object of his cruelty. The sexist, arrogant, greasy-looking man is ogling the hardworking and not-too-attractive lower-middle-class woman he plans to harass. The proud prom queen tries to hide the nail file she was using until the moment the sergeant appeared.

Of course, by the end of the film, these very different people have all grown through their experiences. The black man saves the life of the now contrite racist. The humble woman has quietly and secretly helped the sexist overcome the overwhelming fear that had him crying like a baby. The athlete has learned teamwork. The prom queen has learned to enjoy getting dirty, and the fat guy can now do a hundred pull-ups. Each individual has achieved a basic level of knowledge, adopted a common set of values, and learned an extensive group of skills. As a result, the entire group functions as an effective fighting unit. Boot camp takes a group of individual civilians and puts them through a vigorous and demanding training program to mold them into United States Marines.

Medical training is analogous. People come to medical school from different backgrounds, with different attitudes, and with different levels of medical knowledge. In training, doctors acquire a new set of attitudes and skills that make them able to serve as *physicians*. Like boot camp, the process is difficult and at times seems impossible. Unlike boot camp, medical training lasts seven to fourteen years after the recruit has finished college.

Medical School: The First Two Years

The first day of medical school, as I walked into an air-conditioned lecture hall, the people around me were a lot more homogeneous than the fresh recruits at Parris Island. In part, this is because medical training begins before medical school. To be accepted, we had spent four years in college taking a lot of science courses and getting good grades. Admissions committees like candidates who give back to their community. Therefore, most of my classmates had been active in extracurricular activities, at least some of which were truly service oriented. The final big hurdle to medical school admission is the interview process. Most of my classmates, therefore, were people who made a good first impression.

After we sat down in the big lecture hall, we received a schedule for the rest of the year. Each page covered one week and indicated what classes would be held at each hour. As I flipped through the pages, I choked down the sour taste of acid that had risen in my throat. Classes each day ran from 8 or 9 a.m. to 4 or 5 p.m., except on Fridays when the day usually ended at noon. I had already purchased ten textbooks, each containing at least nine hundred pages. When would I be able to read those and study what I heard in lectures? I also saw that each week was a little different, so that there would never be a weekly routine. I would have to use this daily schedule as my "orders" to tell me what to do; I could not rely on a pattern.

Because I am a morning person, I got up early enough each day to study for an hour or two before attending the morning classes. A group of us would go to lunch together, then back to class or lab for the afternoon. After classes were over, most of us would take a break to go for a run or take a nap. After supper in the cafeteria, each recruit would hide in his or her chosen study location, in the library or at home. A friend down the hall had a television, and a group of us would congregate there every night at 11:30 to enjoy a rerun of the television series *MASH* before going to bed. While most of us took some time off on the weekends, we also spent a lot of weekend time studying.

In most medical schools, the first two years are heavily classroom oriented. The recruit has to memorize a lot of basic scientific principles before she has a chance to understand and practice medicine. In addition to facts, we recruits learn a valuable lesson. The tests that we took were designed to generate a range of scores to distinguish between the smart and smartest. The highest score in the class might be 80 percent. This standard was particularly shocking to a group of people accustomed to getting 90 percent or higher throughout college. The tests were written with the assumption that we knew the concepts and tested whether we knew the details. At the time, I thought that this was cruel, but I now know that knowing the details is essential to being a good doctor. In this educational process, we learned that great sacrifice is absolutely necessary to excel as a physician. Our goal, unobtainable as it might be, was *to know everything about medicine.*

The Clinical Years: Two Days in the Life of a Medical Student

Tuesday, 4:45 a.m.: I arrive on 11 West for another day. Into my white coat's pockets I have stuffed my stethoscope, reflex hammer, penlight, two paperback reference books, various papers and index cards, and a plastic case containing my scopes for looking into ears and eyes. At night when I take it off, I realize that the coat probably weighs about ten pounds.

I find the medical chart on my first patient and look through it. Mrs. Richardson is a forty-five-year-old woman who came to the hospital with a ruptured appendix. When an appendix ruptures before surgery, a lot of infected material gets into the belly. Her initial surgery went well, but because of the infection, her original incision ruptured, and she now has an open wound that is healing from the inside out.

There are no new orders in Mrs. Richardson's chart. The last note in the doctor's section is the note that I, a third-year medical student, had written the day before, duly countersigned by the physicians who are supervising me. I obtain a sterile kit from the nurses' station and take it to Mrs. Richardson's room.

"Good morning, Mrs. Richardson. How are you this morning?"

"I'm fine, just a little sore."

"Did you have any problems overnight?"

"No. None at all."

I lean over and place my stethoscope on her chest. "The heart sounds fine. Just sit up a moment so I can listen to your lungs. Take some deep breaths, in and out, mouth open. That sounds fine also. You can lie down. Let's see how the wound looks."

I open the sterile saltwater solution and pour it into the basin. I remove the outer bandages from her wound, then carefully remove all of the gauze that is packed into it using a long set of forceps (known as tweezers outside the medical world). The bottom layers of gauze are stuck to the dead tissue in the bottom of the wound, and I can pull them away without causing pain. Using a big syringe, I spray 50cc of water into the wound, repeating this process ten times. Mrs. Richardson is quite obese, and the wound is a crater three inches deep and five inches in diameter. Then I moisten new gauze, wringing it out so that it is only a little damp. I repack the wound, finally covering it with a pad of cotton cloth.

"There. How does that feel?"

"It feels fine."

"I know it doesn't seem like you're making much progress, but the wound looks good. It may take months, but eventually it will all heal."

"Thank you, doctor."

Even though I have told Mrs. Richardson that I am a medical student, she, like most of the patients, refers to me as "doctor."

I go back to the nurses' station and place the used supplies where they belong. Then I take her chart and write a note, indicating that she is feeling well, that her examination is as expected, that her labs are OK, and that we will continue with dressing changes and antibiotics.

I go through a similar process with the four other patients I am following, two of whom also require dressing changes. Mrs. Jones had a fever last night that we need to figure out. Mr. Smith's kidney function has deteriorated a little. Mrs. Rittenhouse is slightly tender on the side of the abdomen opposite her incision. I record these new problems in my notes and indicate my plan to deal with them.

Tuesday, 6 a.m.: I meet the intern (in his first year out of medical school) in the hallway by the nurses' station. He has been seeing the patients who do not have a student assigned and has also checked up on the patients I am following, but more briefly. We get a cart and load up the charts of the fifteen patients whom our team is following. The third-year resident (in his third year out of medical school) arrives, and we begin to make rounds together, discussing each patient. We see and examine each patient briefly as a team. The resident tells us what needs to be done for the new problems, adding to or taking away from what we have written in our notes to reflect his plans for the patients. By 7:45 a.m., we have seen the fifteen patients on our service as a team.

Tuesday, 8 a.m.: Now I head to the operating room. Two days ago, Phillip Jones came to the emergency room with nausea and vomiting. His x-rays had shown bowel obstruction, and his CT scan showed a colon cancer. A forty-eight-year-old father of three, he is a hardworking electrical engineer. I stand beside the surgeon who removes the cancerous part of Mr. Jones's colon. My job is to hold retractors (tools to keep other body parts out of the way so the surgeon can see what he is doing) in the right positions for as long as necessary. Sometimes I am called upon to place a stitch, tie a surgical knot, or trim away extra suture after the surgeon has placed a stitch. At 11:30, we move the patient off the operating table onto a bed and take him to the recovery room. I sit down with the resident, and he dictates the postoperative orders as I write them in the chart. These orders give the nurses instructions on how to care for the patient. I don't have much time to reflect on the fact that I have just looked inside the body of a man I met two days ago, but I do feel a few moments of awe.

Tuesday, noon: For the first time in a week, I have time to run by the hospital sandwich shop to grab something to eat on my way to the noon conference. The conference today is about new surgical techniques in gall bladder surgery and is given by a visiting professor. Of course I don't know much about the *old* surgical techniques, but I still learn quite a bit about both by listening. At 12:45, before the lecture is over, I get a page. The resident asks me to come down to the emergency room.

Tuesday, 1 p.m.: When I arrive in the emergency room, the resident sends me to "do a history and physical" on Carl Sinclair. That means that I listen to the story of his illness, ask him enough questions to ensure that I know his entire medical history, do a complete physical examination, review his labs and x-ray tests, and then record all of that information, as well as what I believe his problems and their solutions to be, for inclusion in his chart.

Carl is a twenty-year-old college student who developed abdominal pain about twelve hours ago. Three hours ago, he developed fever, nausea, and vomiting. When I listen to his abdomen, it is silent. Although laypeople talk about their "stomach growling" when they are hungry, medical people know that if you listen to the abdomen with a stethoscope, you normally hear that same noise all the time, just not as loud. A silent abdomen means that something bad is going on. As I touch Carl's abdomen, I discover that he is tender everywhere, but the tenderness is worst in the right lower part of his abdomen. I go out to talk with the resident.

"What do you think?"

"Looks like a classic case of appendicitis."

"That's good, Steve. Go write it up, and then go with him to surgery."

Tuesday, 3 p.m.: I take my "history and physical" up to the operating room and place it in the chart, which is sitting on the anesthesia machine at the head of the operating table. The anesthesiologist has just put Carl to sleep. I like the smell of the iodine in the soap that I use to cleanse my hands and arms as I prepare for surgery. After donning the surgical gown and gloves, I hold retractors as directed and observe the surgery while the surgeon quizzes me about anatomy, appendicitis, and surgical techniques. We finish the postoperative orders at about 5, and I head to the surgical conference room, where "sign-out rounds" are starting.

Tuesday, 5 p.m.: There are three teams like mine on the eleventh-floor surgery division, each with about fifteen patients. Everyone gets a list of the forty-five patients in the division. The resident on each team briefly reviews the condition of the fifteen patients on his service. Only one team is on call each night, and this on-call team has to know about all the patients on the other services in order to handle emergencies that come up. When we finish sign-out rounds at 6:30, the other teams go home, and my team stays. The intern and I grab a quick dinner in the cafeteria. He then sends me to do histories and physicals on two new patients on our service.

One of them, Susie Cohen, is an elderly woman with breast cancer. Ordinarily, she would have come in the following morning for surgery, but she came in with nausea and vomiting two days ago and stayed in the hospital since her surgery was already scheduled for tomorrow.

Karen Johnson, the other patient I see, is a thirty-five-year-old alcoholic admitted with nausea and vomiting due to inflammation of the pancreas—a common affliction of alcoholics. The treatment is to put a tube through the nose into the stomach to suck out all of the liquids so that the intestine is at complete rest. The tube stays in for several days until the pancreas can heal. Ms. Johnson says that she is willing to enter an alcohol rehab program when she is well enough. (Unfortunately, when it comes time for her to go to rehab a week later, she will insist on leaving the hospital with her alcoholic boyfriend instead.)

While I am admitting these two patients, the intern is admitting four others, while answering pages every few minutes about the other forty-five patients in the hospital. I page the intern at 10:30 p.m. and ask if there is anything else I can do to help. He sends me to start an IV on one patient and draw labs on two others. I finish these tasks at 11:15. He then tells me to go on to bed. I am happy to do so, and turn out the light in the call room at 11:25.

Wednesday, 2 a.m.: "BEEEP! BEEEP!" My pager awakens me. I call the number, and the resident asks me to come to the emergency room to see a patient. It is a forty-year-old woman with fever, nausea, vomiting, and abdominal pain. I take her history and examine her. She has profound tenderness under her right rib cage. I discuss the case with the resident, who agrees that this is acute inflammation of the gallbladder. We start her on antibiotics in the hope that surgery can be done in a few days, after the inflammation has settled down.

I crawl back into bed at 3:30. At 4:15 I get up again to take a quick shower and shave.

Wednesday, 4:45 a.m.: I am back on 11 West and go to see Mrs. Richardson, as I did twenty-four hours ago. Today I see six patients before rounds. Some of yesterday's patients have gone home, and four of my patients are the ones I did histories and physicals on in the past twenty-four hours. Our service is bigger now since we took call for the past twenty-four hours: we are up to twenty patients. We still manage to finish rounds as a team by 7:55, and at 8 a.m., having downed two cups of coffee but no breakfast, I am in the operating room with Ms. Cohen for her mastectomy. I dutifully hold the retractors as directed while the surgeon quizzes me about the latest medical and surgical treatments for breast cancer. Fortunately, when I admitted Ms. Cohen, I read about this topic in one of the surgical textbooks. When we finish her postoperative orders at 10 a.m., I stay with the same surgeon to assist in a mastectomy on a patient who came in this morning for elective surgery. As soon as we finish, I head off to the noon conference as soon as we finish; I stop to get a sandwich and arrive at the conference at 12:20.

Wednesday, 1 p.m.: Since I was on call last night, I do not get called today with new admissions. After the conference, I go back to 11 West to check on our patients. I talk with the intern and get a list of x-rays to review. In radiology, I review the films with the radiologist. There are a total of ten patients with x-ray studies. I learn about what can be seen on these x-rays as the radiologist explains the findings. As we discuss the patients, the information on the x-rays helps me to understand what is going on. Mrs. Parker, for example, had a fever this morning. Unfortunately, her chest x-ray shows that her fever is from pneumonia. I take all of this information back to the intern. After we discuss the results, I write notes in the charts, outlining the x-ray findings, and write orders to implement the plans we have made. Between 4 and 5, we discuss each patient with the resident.

Wednesday, 5 p.m.: Sign-out rounds start at 5, and tonight we finish at 6:15. I head for home, where I fall into bed at 8:30 after a quick dinner.

Thursday, 3 a.m.: I get up at 3 a.m. to be at the hospital again at 4:45, where Mrs. Richardson is expecting me. On this rotation, we are on call every third night. Since I took call on Tuesday night, I am not on call again until Friday. Therefore, today I work only from 4:45 a.m. until 6:30 p.m.

On Friday I will be on call again, so I will work from 4:45 a.m. on Friday until Saturday when we finish sign-out rounds. Since there are no elective cases on Saturday, we do sign-out rounds at 11 a.m. All the interns still have to come in on Sunday, but we medical students don't have to come in on Saturday or Sunday unless we are on call. But on Monday morning, I will be back at 4:45 a.m., and I will be at the hospital until 6:30 p.m. on Tuesday.

Clinical Training Overview

After the six-week general surgery rotation, I certainly had a good idea what my remaining years of clinical training would be like. The third year of medical school is spent on rotations like general surgery, working with residents who are doing their training in the various specialties of medicine. Most of the rotations were like the surgery rotation, with a lot of time in the hospital and a little time seeing outpatients. In some specialties, we did not take call in the hospital at all and spent more time seeing outpatients.

The fourth year of medical school was spent taking elective training in areas of medicine where we felt we needed more education. Many of these electives had little inpatient call. Most fourth-year students also spent at least one month as a "subintern," essentially functioning as an intern but with a little more supervision.

The experience of internship (the first year after medical school) is like the surgery rotation described above, except that it is much harder as an intern than it is as a medical student. There is an incredible workload and even more sleep deprivation. Even though my internship program was mostly every fourth night, one of our rotations, the Cardiac Intensive Care Unit, was every other night on call. The pattern on this rotation was that we would come in at about 6 or 6:30 a.m. and see all of our patients. We would then work until about 1 p.m. the next day, and then we would be able to go home until the following morning. We often got no sleep at all during the night on call, so we would go home and sleep most of the hours remaining until we had to go back.

The sleep deprivation of medical training is better now than it was then, due to new regulations. The maximum work week is supposed to be eighty hours. Continuous primary responsibility for patient care is not to exceed twenty-four hours, with an additional six hours are allowed for transfer of responsibility.

Of course, this is still not exactly a cakewalk.

Is there a reason for the sleep deprivation? While the system developed this way largely for historical reasons, there are a number of arguments for its continuation. It certainly teaches self-sacrifice. To some extent, it teaches doctors to function when they are tired, although it also increases medical errors. It allows a lot of medical training to be packed into a smaller number of years. Of course, it also provides hospitals with a source of cheap labor.

Each year after internship gets a little easier. In my program, the second and third year residents had similar call schedules to the interns, but the intern was the one who received the first call when a patient had a problem. As a resident, my calls were either about new patients needing to be admitted to the hospital or from an intern when she or he needed help with a problem.

All of medical training is characterized by graduated responsibility. As a beginning medical student, everything I did was supervised. As I learned to do simple tasks, like drawing blood or starting an IV, I did these things independently. As the years go by, trainees do more advanced procedures independently, from physical examinations to sophisticated surgeries. This progression continues throughout medical training, with each trainee growing professionally as she proves herself to her superiors.

In addition to the clinical work, there is a lot of book learning. Reading textbooks, looking up new papers in the medical literature, reading the latest journals, and studying for national examinations are all a part of the training years.

Clinical training after medical school can last anywhere from three to ten years, depending on the specialty and the institution. The top programs in the country usually require one to three years of research, often in the laboratory, in addition to clinical training. Some specialties, like cardiology and surgical fields, are heavily inpatient and require a lot of call in the hospital throughout training. Other fields, like dermatology and family practice, are heavily outpatient and have much less inpatient call after the internship year.

Clinical Training Values

Throughout these years of training, doctors are under continual scrutiny by those both above and below them in the training program. Our superiors expected us to know everything about each patient and their medical problems, and we expected the same of ourselves. Failure to do something that needed to be done was unacceptable. That an action was difficult, or even impossible, was not an acceptable excuse. We would make whatever sacrifice was necessary for our patients. Being tired, sleepless, hungry, dirty, or unshaven was no reason not to go the extra mile to fully evaluate and treat every problem, and indeed to do whatever constituted a full evaluation, even if it was not obviously related to the problem the patient was having. When an intern in my program told his resident that he had not done the rectal exam on his new patient, he was informed—with a smile but also as a definite warning—that there were only two reasons not to do a rectal exam: (1) no finger or (2) no rectum.

While I want to communicate how intensely grueling this experience is, I also want you to see that there is something incredibly gratifying about the intensity of training. The privilege of being intimately involved in so many lives and in so many critical decisions in each twenty-four-hour day is sometimes exhilarating, especially when we have the chance to save a life. Surviving the demands, saving the patients, and sharing these experiences build the identity of being a doctor.

Bear in mind that call responsibilities do not end after training. In the scenarios described above, I refer to teaching hospitals, where there are interns and residents staffing all the hospital services. Most hospitals nationally do not have interns or residents. Therefore, when the nurse has a question or concern, he or she calls the attending physician, a doctor who has completed training and is now in private practice. If the patient needs to be seen or requires a procedure, the doctor comes to the hospital to provide the needed service.

There are no legal limits on the hours of attending physicians. The hours that an attending physician works are dictated by a combination of choices and necessities. Attending physicians have a responsibility to ensure that care is available to their patients at all times. They arrange coverage of their patients with each other by mutual agreement. When working and providing call coverage, the attending physician is available twenty-four hours a day. For many physicians, that responsibility continues for days or even weeks at a time. Fortunately, it does not mean staying constantly in the hospital, and it does not usually mean being up all night, although that potential always exists. For physicians who care for critically ill patients, the time demands are most severe. In contrast, there are physicians who have a strictly outpatient practice, and they may provide no after-hours coverage. Thus there is a broad spectrum of degrees of time demand, but most doctors have some degree of call responsibility throughout their entire career.

Results of Training

This process of training inculcates certain traits, both positive and negative, in the individuals who persevere through it. One of the strongest and most important traits is *responsibility*. The doctor is the individual responsible for every aspect of the patient's care. The intern is expected to have all of the tests available for the attending physician. If that means harassing the medical records department repeatedly for hours, then that is what is expected. If it means breaking into the radiology department to steal the films that the technician can't find, then that is expected as well. It is the tradition of the *MASH* television series, where battling against bureaucracies for the sake of patients was an art form. Responsibility means that there is no excuse for providing inadequate care. "I was too tired" is never an acceptable answer. "I did not think of that possibility" is also not acceptable. The doctor is expected to think of every possibility and do every appropriate test *before* being asked by a superior. The system encourages doctors to strive for excellence and a superhuman perfection against impossible working conditions.

A second related trait is *self-sacrifice*. I am expected to sacrifice personal comfort in the form of sleep and relaxation beginning before medical school and continuing throughout my career, in order to provide the best possible care to my patients. Self-sacrifice also translates into family sacrifice. If my patient is having a heart attack, I cannot continue the needed conversation with my wife or children at that time. We routinely reschedule family birthdays to ensure an uninterrupted celebration. While this is not an ideal situation for my family, it is unavoidable in my profession.

A third positive trait encouraged by physician training is *hard work*. As detailed above, the workload throughout training is heavy. A physician who succeeds learns to work hard and efficiently and to accept responsibility readily. Seeking out new information needed to help a patient should be automatic. Going in at night when needed should be done without hesitation.

A fourth positive trait is *camaraderie* with fellow physicians. Those of us who have endured this process have a sense of understanding with other physicians that those who have not been through it cannot share. Our high regard for one another and our understanding of each other leads to immediate mutual accessibility. I can telephone the office of any physician in the country and simply state that I am Dr. Brown calling for Dr. Whomever, and I will be put through immediately. Patients generally have no idea how much consultation occurs in this manner as we seek to provide quality health care. We routinely discuss with radiologists what tests need to be done or what their results are. We frequently have extended conversations about patients with consultants, to determine how best to care for them. Our camaraderie with each other facilitates the delivery of complex modern health care. It also provides us with comfort in working with each other in the face of powerful stresses in our lives as the practice of medicine becomes more impersonal and difficult.

Unfortunately, the training process also encourages the development of some negative traits. One of the earliest, which hopefully the physician outgrows, is a *survival mentality*. The pressures on the intern are so profound, and the year of sleep deprivation is so painful, that the primary goal of the intern is simply to survive. Survival requires hard work and self-sacrifice, but it also requires conserving energy and sleeping and resting whenever possible. The natural effort to conserve energy ends up limiting one's investment of time and emotional energy in other pursuits. It may mean sacrificing family desires and responsibilities and allowing others to fulfill responsibilities outside work that are really one's own. To some extent, a doctor's spouse always ends up with extra work due to the unique nature of medical responsibilities. The survival mentality sometimes extends into the medical workplace, with interns dumping their work on other interns. Although the internship

A Christian Perspective

In Matthew 20, Jesus says, "Whoever desires to be great among you, let him be your servant. And whoever desires to be first among you, let him be your slave—just as the Son of Man did not come to be served, but to serve, and to give His life as a ransom for many." The self-sacrificial servanthood exemplified by Jesus is the goal of the ideal physician. When I am on call for my group, if anyone among the 250,000 people in the drawing area of our hospital has a heart attack, I am her servant for the next several hours until she is treated and stabilized. I give up control of my schedule to sacrifice myself, my interests, and my comfort to the needs of those I am serving. This is true servanthood, in the best possible sense.

What about doctors who do not share my Christian beliefs? Most doctors of all belief systems value the self-sacrifice and devotion that are inculcated in our training. The vast majority make great sacrifices on a regular basis to help their patients. Even though they may not have a Christian basis for these sacrifices, they share the same ideal of selfless duty to their patients.

year is the hardest year, some doctors maintain that same survival mentality throughout their life. The survival mentality may be perceived by others as pride or selfishness, but the underlying motivation is usually the physician's desperation to hold together incompatible responsibilities. Unfortunately, even though this mentality is not intentional cruelty, its victims are hurt as badly as if it were.

A second bad attitude encouraged by the training is *pride*. Knowing that he has gone through such an impossible period of training may make the doctor feel entitled to better treatment in other spheres or to feel generally superior to others. Pride can also be manifested in a lack of compassion for others. It can be a self-centered attitude that expects others to make the sacrifices necessary to allow the doctor to continue to avoid her responsibilities outside the medical practice, even when she could fulfill them herself.

A third negative effect of training is *emotional coldness*. I still remember vividly that about six months after I finished my internship, my attitudes toward others changed perceptibly. I looked back on events that had happened at the end of internship and thought about how I had responded emotionally. I could now see that my attitudes were not compassionate, even though at the time they had seemed reasonable. I could finally see through eyes that were not so sleep deprived. I had a much healthier perspective on relationships. Sadly, some doctors never regain a healthy perspective but continue to be cold toward patients.

The Culmination of Training

The best possible outcome of training is a doctor who is responsible, self-sacrificing, knowledgeable, skilled, tireless, and hardworking. He has overcome the pride and survival mentality that characterized the early years of training and is now mature and compassionate, with the patient's best interests paramount over all other concerns. Like the recruits at Parris Island who become ideal marines, the trainee has now become the ideal doctor.

Doctors aspire to this goal, and most practice in a way that reflects it. We evaluate each other by our adherence to this standard, and you should try to evaluate us by the same standard.

Choosing a Physician

How can we use this understanding of medical training and standards to choose the best possible physician? We can seek a doctor who exemplifies the qualities of an ideal physician, as exemplified by the standards of our training.

1. *Find a physician who exemplifies self-sacrifice.* A person's character is reflected in all areas of their work. Because of that, you do not have to wait until you are critically ill to assess your doctor's character. His or her character will be evident in little things.

If you need a physician whose specialty involves caring for many critically ill people in the hospital (such as a heart doctor, lung doctor, stomach doctor, or surgeon), try to befriend a nurse or clerk who works in the emergency room or critical care unit, and ask them who calls back quickly when they are paged. Doctors who care about their patients want to know when they are developing a problem that the nurse feels requires their attention. You would be amazed at how much variation there is in promptness, with some doctors calling back in seconds while others do not call back at all even after several pages. The nurses know who responds promptly and who does not. Reports from other patients about sacrifice are good clues to character as well. Self-sacrifice is also evident in how well the doctor demonstrates the other qualities listed below.

2. *Choose a doctor who demonstrates thoroughness.* I mentioned earlier that during training, doctors are taught to fully assess every patient, even in areas not directly related to the immediate problem. When you first see a new doctor, do they try to learn about all of your past history, or do they only focus on the problem that led to the visit? A thorough doctor should ask about other medical problems, either verbally or through a questionnaire. If done through a questionnaire, they should look at the questionnaire, and ask for additional details when the answers are not clear. If you are seeing a doctor for primary care, they should do a thorough examination, not only of the area of concern but also of the rest of your body. If they cannot do so due to time constraints on your first visit, they should say so, and arrange for a "complete physical" at a later date. This thoroughness should be provided no matter how knowledgeable you seem to be about your health.

Several years ago, a fellow physician came to me for a checkup. As is my custom, I asked him all the important questions about his past history. A week later, he sent me a gift along with a card that said, "Thank you for treating me like a *patient.*"

Sometimes you are not able to choose your physician. In that situation, you can gently insist on thoroughness. A couple of years ago, a patient of mine went to the emergency room with a cough and fever. She was diagnosed with bronchitis, but the physician who saw her did not listen to her lungs. Later, she saw her primary care physician, who discovered that she had pneumonia. If the physician who first saw her had listened to her lungs, he might have reached the correct diagnosis. Failure to listen to the lungs of a patient with cough and fever is malpractice. When you find yourself in this unfortunate situation, it is OK to say something like "I would really feel better if you listened to my lungs." Sometimes, believe it or not, doctors get sidetracked and forget that they haven't done an appropriate examination. But even if they are just lazy, gentle coaxing can encourage better conduct.

3. *Choose a doctor who communicates.* Character is also evident in how you are treated. Does the doctor take the time to answer your questions, or is she only interested in grunting a few syllables and getting you out of the office? A patient once told me that when she went to a particular doctor, she would always sit in front of the door so that he could not easily escape until he had answered her questions. If you have to do this, find another doctor.

Does the doctor explain why she is ordering tests on you? Does she explain the results? Do her explanations make sense? How does she respond, or react, to questions? What does she say when you ask about other options? Is she offended, or does she explain the reasons for her recommendations openly? Find a doctor who cares enough to communicate.

4. *Choose a doctor who demonstrates knowledge.* One thing that distinguishes me from a witch doctor wearing a loincloth and dancing around a fire is the knowledge that I have, based on scientific study, of what treatments work and what treatments do not work. In training, doctors learn to read the latest medical reports with skepticism and to examine them critically to see what they add to current medical knowledge. You should ask your doctor how we know that a particular treatment is better, and your doctor should have an answer. If you have a rare disorder or an unusual situation, it is fine for your doctor to tell you that he needs to do some reading to come up with the

latest information about your health care. If you have a chronic disease, ask from time to time if there are any new findings about that disease. When discussing a proposed test or treatment, your doctor should talk about pros and cons, or should have an answer if you ask about pros and cons. Often you will know without asking any questions how knowledgeable your doctor is by what he tells you and what he asks you.

5. *Protect yourself using the principles discussed in chapter 2.* Take any clues that suggest bad character very seriously, before it is too late. Most states have information about health-care practitioners on the website of their licensing entity, often called the state medical board. While a disciplinary action may not necessarily mean a bad doctor, you should at least avail yourself of the information there and consider it in the context of your other observations. Often the details of any disciplinary actions are available for you to make your own assessment.

Conclusion

Most doctors are of good character and try to do the best for their patients. However, using the guidelines above, you should seek out a doctor who is not just good but outstanding. In the next chapter, I will discuss how to support your chosen doctor and how to build a strong relationship to make your health care both pleasant and thorough.

4

✚

Support Your Local Doctor

"Dr. Brown," Julie said, "I understand better now the training that you have been through to be a doctor. I want to know how to help you take better care of me and how to support you and my other doctors. What stresses do you face now, and how can I encourage you?"

"Julie, it's kind of you to ask that question. I'm happy to answer it."

Gratefulness

I finally finished seeing the last patient in the office for the afternoon. Earlier in the day, I had had to rush to the hospital twice for emergencies, and most of the office patients had opted to wait rather than to reschedule. I looked at my desk, piled high with charts in which I would now

have to do my paperwork. Off to the side, on top of my
mail, was a small envelope that was hand addressed. I
opened it and removed the card inside.

> Dear Dr. Brown,
>   Thank you so much for coming in at 2 o'clock in the
> morning to take care of Bill with his heart attack. We know
> that you have a family of your own, and we appreciate the
> sacrifices that you make for *our* family.
>
> Sincerely,
> Sylvia Johnson

Those two sentences carried me through all of the paperwork. They also created a bond between that family
and me, making it easy to go the extra mile for them the
next time they have a problem.

Your doctor faces a number of different stresses. Some of
them, like having to get up in the middle of the night, are
obvious. Others you may not think about. You can make
your doctor's life easier and more pleasant by understanding the problems he faces in the practice of medicine. By
making his life easier, you will get better medical care.

Failure

Most people die in a hospital, and most of them die
despite their doctor's best efforts. Doctors are fallible, and
medical science also fails: many problems are not curable.
When a patient dies or has a bad outcome, it is always
disturbing to the family—and to the doctor.

When a death or bad outcome is expected, the patient,
the family, and the doctor often grow closer through the
experience. The doctor discusses with the patient and the
family what to expect and ensures that the patient is kept
comfortable, even if his death is inevitable. Many patients

have chosen me as their doctor because they remember how kind I was to their Uncle Fred when he was dying a few years before.

On the other hand, when a death or bad outcome is unexpected, no one is emotionally prepared, and it is very difficult for the family to cope. More than you might think, it is also hard for the doctor. Unanswered questions and guilt hang over the scene like clouds, ready to afflict everyone with the rain of grief and the lightning of blame. Often the air could be cleared completely by a talk between a family member and the doctor. Just call the doctor's office and explain to a nurse that you have some questions about what happened to your loved one and would like to sit down and talk about what happened or even to speak with the doctor on the telephone. This type of conversation will be therapeutic for you and also for the doctor involved. It will also probably put your mind at ease. Instead of giving you the answers, it may reveal that the answers are not known. If there are no answers, it will still be helpful for you and the doctor to grieve together.

The Malpractice Crisis

The most painful experience that a doctor can have professionally is to be sued for malpractice. Because of our training, our role as doctor is central to our identity. We expect perfection of ourselves, and the suggestion that we have failed in our duties is a blow to the core of our being.

The doctor will have great fear, even if she is innocent, that a jury will not understand the complexities of the science. In a malpractice suit, the doctor is not facing a jury of her peers but a jury of laypeople with no medical background. Even if her conduct was perfect, a jury may not understand.

The lack of honesty in our society interferes with the legal process. It is now possible to find a medical expert who will testify to anything. Too often, families also do not tell the truth in a case. Our legal system depends on people's telling the truth under oath. Since in our society truth telling is no longer a controlling value, there is no way the legal system can do what it is supposed to do. The medical system places a great deal of importance on telling the truth about what happened. Discovering that this value is no longer universal in the legal system is a painful source of frustration to doctors.

During the time between the filing of a lawsuit and a trial, which can extend anywhere from a year to many years, the doctor is continually distracted by it. He cannot provide the same quality of care due to this continual distraction. He tends to practice medicine defensively for the rest of his life, doing more tests and being less forthcoming with patients about his actual opinions than he had been before. The lawsuit takes a tremendous emotional toll on the doctor and his family, and it causes his patients to suffer as well.

When a doctor is sued, especially if she did nothing wrong, it invariably causes her to consider discontinuing the practice of medicine. Good doctors who have been in practice for a significant length of time know that they would be just as happy making less money. They have been making great sacrifices for their patients, and these sacrifices are affecting their families. When such sacrifices are met with the ungratefulness of a lawsuit, a doctor asks herself why she is subjecting herself to this suffering.

Many malpractice suits originate because of a misunderstanding of the medical issues by the patient's family, particularly after an unexpected bad outcome. In many cases, instead of going to the doctor for answers, the family will simply obtain medical records and will misinterpret some of the information. If they consult a plaintiff's attorney, the attorney has a vested interest in pursuing the case rather than explaining the issues to the family. In the few legal cases I have reviewed, the family's misunderstanding invariably contributed to the decision to sue.

Usually, even if an error was made, the doctor was doing the best he knew to do for the patient, but the family is led to believe that the doctor did not care. The jury is hammered hard with the same view if the case goes to trial. Flagrant disregard for a patient does happen, but it is rare. There are certainly doctors who deserve to be sued, but there are more who are sued despite their best efforts. Often the doctors who *deserve* to be sued fool their victims completely.

If you decide that you want to initiate a lawsuit against a physician, find the best malpractice lawyer you can by getting a referral from another attorney. Do *not* go to someone because he or she has placed an ad on television. The most successful lawyers, like the most successful physicians, do not need to advertise. A successful attorney is more likely to give you an honest appraisal of the situation. If he or she tells you that you do not have a case, you are probably getting an honest opinion. Ask the attorney the questions you have about the case, and you may get your misunderstandings cleared up. On the other hand, if an already successful attorney does take your case, it is more likely that the case is appropriate.

From a public policy standpoint, lawsuits do not lead doctors to practice better medicine. Further, when the bills for defense are paid, the money does not come from the guilty doctor. Most of the money is paid by the insurance company, which passes the bill on to all of its policyholders, who pass the bill on to the recipients of health care, and sooner or later that group includes everyone. So the punishment for the guilty is no greater than the punishment for the innocent. Lawsuits also result in less availability of health care, as doctors migrate to areas with a better malpractice environment and retire earlier than they would otherwise.

Complaining about a case to the hospital's peer review committee or your state's medical board stands a better chance of identifying real problems and generating real solutions. Unfortunately, the actions of these entities are also legal proceedings. In the case of state medical boards, there has been growing political pressure to discipline more people, and this has resulted in some inappropriate actions. On the other hand, the system sometimes errs in favor of protecting the rights of the physician instead of the public. However, at least these organizations exist in a medical context, where the chances of an accurate decision are higher. Moreover, their power allows them to sanction the individual physician involved.

Your doctor will not tell you that he is in the midst of a lawsuit or that he has been through a lawsuit. However, the possibility of lawsuits is always there. You encourage your doctor by showing appreciation for his efforts and by asking questions in a nonjudgmental way when you have a bad outcome. You also help yourself and your family by staying informed about the risks and limitations of therapies and tests, so that you are not surprised unnecessarily if a bad outcome occurs.

Nonadherence

Nonadherence is a medical term that refers to a patient's failure to follow the doctor's advice. Now you may think to yourself, "What does the doctor care? Her job is to give advice, and she gets paid the same whether her patients accept it or not." On unimportant issues, I suppose this is true. However, most of the issues I deal with relate to helping people live longer and preventing heart attacks and strokes. I care about my patients, so it bothers me to see them make bad decisions. Often people do not follow my advice because they overestimate the risks of taking their medications and underestimate the risks of not taking them. Sometimes they just forget or fail to pay attention to instructions. At other times they cannot afford their medications but are embarrassed to tell me that, even though I can often help with this problem. Whatever the reason, my inability to help people because of nonadherence is frustrating.

Nonadherence is also a legal liability issue. When a patient dies from not following the doctor's advice, sometimes the family will still sue the physician, claiming that he or she did not do enough to get the patient to comply.

If for some reason you do not wish to follow a doctor's advice, you need to have a frank discussion with the doctor about your concerns. Usually, the concerns that people have are a result of their lack of knowledge. In some cases, your concerns may be completely valid, and the doctor will discuss the reason for recommending the therapy despite those concerns. Sometimes after such a discussion, the doctor may accept your decision not to follow his advice. Not following the doctor's advice without such a discussion would have cheated you of the benefit of the doctor's expertise and frustrated the doctor with your unexplained actions, which then appear due to carelessness on your part. More important, such a discussion is necessary for an honest relationship.

Sometimes when a patient refuses to comply with the doctor's advice, the patient will be "fired" or dismissed from the doctor's practice. Doctors, in general, have a legal right to choose not to treat whomever they wish, for any reason (with the exception of reasons that are discriminatory) or for no reason, with or without explanation. By far the most common reason I dismiss patients is for a failure to follow my advice, usually after multiple warnings. Their failure may be deliberate (they do not wish to do what I recommend), or it may be due to failure to come in for follow-up as directed. In either of these situations, their continued follow-up with me would be a waste of my time and their money. They should be seeing a doctor whose advice they *will* follow. To dismiss a patient, the doctor is obligated to give reasonable notice to the patient and to ensure continuity of care by giving the patient directions for obtaining care from a different physician.

Physician Shortages

Another source of stress for your physician is the shortage of doctors. A few years ago, there were predictions that health maintenance organizations (HMOs) would dominate the world of healthcare. No matter how serious your health problem might be, you would have to go to your primary care doctor first. Primary care doctors would treat the vast majority of problems, with only a few patients being sent on to specialists. However, these predictions were wrong, mainly because those enrolled in HMOs insisted on freer access to specialists. But when the predictions were made, the government gave medical schools incentives to produce larger percentages of primary care physicians, and money was allocated to increase the number of primary care residency positions. As a result, many new medical school graduates went into primary care fields instead of other medical specialties.

In cardiology, the results have been disastrous. The baby boomers are now aging and developing heart disease. Studies have shown better outcomes when cardiologists rather than primary care doctors provide care after heart attacks. Cardiology procedures such as angioplasty are becoming more effective and more widely used. The result is a terrible shortage of cardiologists nationally. The same thing is true in many other areas of medicine. The shortages are aggravated by the early retirement of many doctors, who make this choice because of the time stresses, the malpractice crisis, declining reimbursement, and the increasing bureaucracy associated with practicing medicine. Because of the shortages, most good doctors are overworked.

Because of being overworked, wise doctors establish boundaries. For example, a patient recently complained to me that her brother's cardiologist would not prescribe a medicine for him to stop smoking. My patient thought that this was terrible, because I had given medicine to her for that purpose. As I explained to my patient, we all have to limit what we do. While I had chosen to prescribe medicine to help her stop smoking, the cardiologist caring for her brother has chosen to leave that therapy in the hands of her brother's primary care physician. To prescribe a medication requires understanding the potential side effects, the interactions with other drugs, and the available alternatives when the medicine does not work. It may look like no big deal to you as the recipient of the therapy, but it is a big deal that becomes a lot bigger when multiplied by the many patients who will receive it. When your doctor establishes a boundary, you should respect it. Not only will this help your doctor, it protects you from receiving therapy from someone who would be only marginally qualified to provide it.

Boundaries are also important in terms of access. Do not call your doctor at home unless you have his or her permission. In general, you should contact the answering service after hours and on weekends. Your doctor may be in town but may have someone else taking her calls so that she can have time with her family. Call after hours or on a weekend only if you believe you have a medical emergency. (If you come into the hospital with a heart attack, you do not want your doctor being interrupted because someone else needs a prescription refill.) If you already know that you or your loved one will need to be seen, there is no need to call: just go to the hospital emergency room, where the emergency-room doctor can initiate the evaluation quickly. In short, treat your doctor the way you would want to be treated by *your* employer.

Reimbursement

Another issue that affects doctors emotionally is payment. I am amazed, and I hope you would be amazed also, at the significant minority of patients who do not pay their doctors. Of course, to accept services and then not pay for them is theft. It is no different from shoplifting. These people may think that the doctor has plenty of money or that Santa Claus or the government pays us for services that we provide free. Unfortunately, while I am comfortable financially, the provision of services not only costs me time but also costs money for all of my ancillary staff. I happily provide many services without charge, but I appreciate the opportunity to make that decision and do not appreciate the deceptiveness of stealing from me.

Most of the time, if a patient or family informs the doctor's office that they cannot afford to pay, the doctor will work out a payment plan that allows them to pay the money gradually, or the doctor may agree to write off the charges entirely. There is certainly no other business that is so sympathetic. The bottom line is to be honest about your situation and discuss options with the doctor. The doctor

A Christian Perspective

In the Bible, Luke, a physician, tells a story in which Jesus heals ten lepers. The lepers cry out to Jesus from a distance, and Jesus responds graciously and tells them to show themselves to the priests, which was the prescribed way to have their healing confirmed so that they could rejoin society. On the way to see the priests, they were healed. One of the ten returns to Jesus and falls down on his face before him, thanking him for the healing. Jesus then asks, "Were there not ten cleansed? But where are the nine?"

I am paid for the work I do as a doctor. I also derive satisfaction for doing a good job whether I am thanked or not. However, far fewer than one in ten patients go out of their way to thank me, beyond the simple thanks at the end of a visit that courtesy requires. A few extra words of thanks mean a lot. A brief thank-you note means more than you can imagine. A little encouragement like this goes a long way and erases a lot of the frustrations of the day. It also makes your doctor closer to you emotionally. That connection means better care and more patience when you have a new problem or need to ask a few more questions than usual.

Finally, you can help tremendously by praying for your doctors and their families. There are a multitude of frustrations and pressures on doctors and their families today. The financial rewards that still exist in medicine mean the least to the doctors who are the best in character, and so these doctors are often the most tempted to retire early. Pray for strength and encouragement. Pray for strong families. Pray for wisdom. And it is also OK to let your doctor know that you appreciate him and are praying for him. Even if he is an atheist, he will appreciate the sentiment.

may offer alternative resources for your care as well. Most communities have clinics that offer free or reduced-cost care. Many of them are staffed by doctors, maybe even your own doctors, who volunteer their time in that setting, where overhead costs may be covered by the county hospital or through other government entities.

Honesty about your ability to afford medications is also imperative. Your doctor can help by providing samples or by giving you information about prescription assistance programs run by the pharmaceutical companies or local organizations in your community. Alternatively, the doctor may prescribe medications that are less expensive. You will find that the doctor will appreciate your candor. Too often a doctor will develop a plan of treatment and then not learn until a follow-up visit that the medications were never taken because the patient could not afford to fill the prescription.

Another financial pressure on your doctor is the fact that reimbursements are not rising as they should to keep pace with inflation and the increasing costs of providing health care. Increases in malpractice premiums, energy costs, labor costs, and computerization are not reimbursed. Instead, declining reimbursements are reflected in declining physician salaries. Realizing that I will make less money next year even though I will do more work is not a pleasant thought. However, most doctors do not go into medicine for the money, and you can make a big difference to our emotional state by expressing your appreciation in other ways.

Summary

So what can you do to support your physician? I have answered this question as we have gone along, but I will review the key points here.

1. Understand that medicine is imperfect. When you or a member of your family has a bad outcome, ask the doctor your questions about what happened and recognize that medicine does not cure all disease.
2. Follow your doctor's advice. When you do not want to do this, discuss the reasons with your doctor.
3. Respect the boundaries set by your physician, and treat her the way you would want to be treated.
4. Pay your doctor what you owe for his services. If you are unable to do so, be honest with him and his office staff about this issue.
5. If you are unable to afford medications, tests, or procedures, tell your doctor. There are usually resources available to help you.
6. Express appreciation to your doctor with words, notes, goodies, and prayers.

Looking Ahead

In part 1, we have examined the world of modern health care by focusing on the doctor. We have seen that there are bad doctors and have discussed how to avoid them. We have looked at health from the doctor's point of view and learned how to find and keep a good doctor. In part 2, we will look at the philosophical underpinnings that have allowed the tremendous advances in health care that have occurred in the past hundred years, and we'll learn how to apply these principles as we make health-care decisions.

PART **2**

✚

THE PRINCIPLES

5

✚

How Do We Know
If a Treatment Works?

"Dr. Brown," Julie continued, "I understand that a lot of medicine is not black and white and that bad things can happen no matter what treatment we choose. I would like to know more about how to evaluate treatments scientifically."

"I am glad that you do. Understanding the issues of medicine will allow you to travel more safely through this maze of health care by looking at the issues for yourself and asking your doctor the right questions. To get you to that point, I need to help you understand how medicine has changed in the past four thousand years. Have you ever heard of bloodletting as a treatment?"

"Isn't that what helped kill George Washington?"

"It certainly didn't help him get well. Bloodletting was a worthless treatment that was practiced from ancient times until a century ago. Changes in the way we think about science finally led to the conclusion that bloodletting should be abandoned as a therapy. Unfortunately, faulty reasoning is still with us today. Being able to recognize good and bad reasoning will help you evaluate advice you hear."

Ancient Rome, 2nd Century

I am Claudius Galenus, and the year is AD 170. I am a physician, and Marcus Gladius has called me to his home to see his wife, Phronesis, who is ill.

"Phronesis, I was so sorry to hear about your illness."

"Claudius, I am most grateful for your concern. I am delighted that the most celebrated physician in the empire is able to see me."

"What has been happening?"

"Two days ago, I started coughing. At first the cough was mild, and nothing came up. Since yesterday, I have been coughing all the time, and thick phlegm has been coming up."

"Did you save some?"

"Yes. Do you want to see it?"

"Of course."

She had the servant bring a cloth that contained the phlegm. It was thick and dark yellow.

"Have you had any other symptoms?"

"Yes. I have had high fever as well. I also haven't felt like eating much."

"Phronesis, how old are you?"

"I am twenty."

Phronesis had the typical symptoms of a condition we call pneumonia. We understand through the work of our philosophers that the body is composed of four humors.

Disease occurs when the humors are out of balance, with excesses or deficiencies of one or more of them. Therefore, the treatment of disease is aimed at getting the humors back in balance. Pneumonia is caused by an excess of phlegm. We know that phlegm is in vomit, so the way to treat pneumonia is to administer medications that cause vomiting. I explained this to Phronesis as gently as I could.

"I understand. My cousin had the same problem and got better after the same treatment."

I spoke with her husband, Marcus, before I left.

"Will she recover?"

"In all probability, yes. Not everyone with pneumonia recovers, but her youth is in her favor."

United States, 21st Century

Where on earth did Claudius get the idea that making people vomit is an effective treatment for pneumonia? Was he crazy? Was he intellectually challenged? What about the idea that the body is made of four humors? Did that idea last very long?

Before we get into these issues specifically, let's step back for a moment and take a panoramic view of history.

A Great Shift

What was life like five hundred years ago compared to five thousand years ago, from a scientific, technological standpoint? What was the fastest form of transportation at either time? That would be riding a horse, wouldn't it? What about climate control? Fires and hand-held fans were all they had. What about medicine? Medicine used ineffective practices like bloodletting. No meaningful progress was made in fifty centuries.

Now compare five hundred years ago to today. Transportation has moved from horseback to supersonic jets. Climate control is the reason you can read this book in relative comfort all year round. Medicine has now moved from bloodletting to routine open-heart surgery.

What changed? Why the explosion of progress in the last five centuries?

The Dogma of Reason and Tradition

Claudius, in the story above, relied on *reason* to understand the world. The ancient Greeks believed that truth is determined using reason. If you thought carefully enough and accurately enough about a problem, you would arrive at the truth. Using reason alone, Hippocrates, the father of medicine, articulated a theory that the body is composed of four humors. Disease results from these humors being out of balance. Effective medical treatments were those that restored the balance of the humors.

The ancients also taught that reality cannot be determined through the physical senses, because the senses can be deceived and because the physical world is only a shadow of the real, spiritual world. If a theory does not seem to correspond to the world that we see, the discrepancy is explained by the fact that human senses are not reliable. And since the human senses are not reliable, there is no reason to do experiments. Observations are irrelevant. Truth has to be determined by careful thought.

The concept that reason is superior to observation was articulated by Plato and developed by Aristotle. In the history of science, this view is called Aristotelianism. Aristotle used reason to write detailed discussions about all sorts of natural phenomena. For example, he discussed the issue of falling objects. He asserted that if two balls were dropped at the same time, the heavier of the balls would fall faster.

He wrote exhaustively about many areas of science. His writings became the basis for scientific thought and remained so for centuries.

Aristotle and the other ancient Greeks were held in high esteem in the centuries that followed. After all, they had explained how to understand the world. Since their theories were carefully reasoned, the world looked back to their writings as authoritative sources for philosophy and science. Thus, *tradition* became the second major source of truth in the world. If Aristotle said it, that settled the argument.

It was impossible to topple the Greek philosophers from their thrones without a fundamental change in philosophy. No one could attack Aristotle or Plato or Hippocrates on the basis that their theory did not correspond to actual observations, since in their philosophy, observation was inferior to reasoning.

France, 15th Century

Father Caché loved the coolness of the stone walls and floors of the monastery in the summertime, but he hated their frigidity in winter. Now fifty years of age, he was one of the oldest monks residing there. He was proud of his monastery's reputation as a place of both learning and healing. Sitting in his study, he wore the gloves that his sister had knitted for him, with the tips of the thumb and two fingers of the right hand uncovered to allow him to write. He shivered anytime a draft came through the room. Huddled by the fireplace in his study, a blanket over his shoulders, he read the works of Plato by the light of the flickering flames. Occasionally, the putrid smell of a chamberpot would waft into the room as the attendant carried it out to the garden from the ward where the patients stayed.

When Brother Decouvert knocked on the door, Father Caché did not stir from his cocoon but instead called out to him. "Come in, François, and close the door behind you. Pull a chair up to the fire. What can I do for you, Brother?"

"Father, I have been thinking and praying about our recent experiences with patients afflicted by pneumonia."

"So have I, François. I have been quite saddened by the fact that we have had five deaths in two weeks."

"Father, all five died shortly after they had been bled."

"Yes. They all worsened shortly after that treatment."

"Father, I wonder if bleeding is as beneficial as the ancients believed."

"François, bleeding has been in use for thousands of years. Of course it is beneficial. Those patients died despite the bleeding. They would have died even sooner without it."

"Why don't we find out? If I may be so bold, I would propose that the next ten patients we have with pneumonia be treated with all of the usual therapies, except without the bleeding, and then the next ten after that with bleeding. We can then compare the groups and see if bleeding helps as much as we have thought."

The older monk shook his head and wondered to himself what they were teaching youth these days.

"François, do you not know the works of Plato?"

"Of course I do, Father."

"Then you understand how misleading the appearance of things in the world can be. To know whether bleeding helps, you need to get a clear conception of the nature of man and the nature of pneumonia, and *reason out* what treatments will help. Doing a test like the one you propose can be very misleading, since the nature of things *can be discerned only in our minds*, not in our bodies. You also know that we need not approach these things on our own. We need to rely on the wisdom of the ancients. If bleeding was good enough for Aristotle and Hippocrates, it is certainly good enough for François Decouvert!"

"Father, I know it sounds arrogant, but I watched young Michael getting better. Then, after each bleeding, he would worsen again. I wanted with all my heart to stop the bleeding."

"Your compassion is to be commended, but you must not let it interfere with your better judgment. Many treatments make our patients feel worse in the short run, but it is not always easy to get the humors back into balance. With the fevers that he had, you know that he had an excess of blood. Let's look at Galen's treatise on pneumonia together."

United States, 21st Century

This view, that truth is determined by reason and tradition, dominated not only medical thought but all of scientific thought for centuries. If two scholars in the Middle Ages had a disagreement about the planets or the human body or the nature of anything, it would not be settled by experiment or observation. Instead, it would be settled by looking back at the writings of the Greek philosophers and employing logic based on their statements.

Because of this worldview, there was no meaningful progress in science or medicine. In the view of Hippocrates and his ancient Greek successors, bloodletting could get the humors back in balance, and therefore it was practiced into the 1800s. Since experimentation was considered worthless and observation was of no value, a true scholar was one who best knew the writings of the ancients.

A New Paradigm

What happened five hundred years ago that allowed scientific progress? In matters scientific, the Renaissance started when scientists questioned the dogma of Aristotle and examined how Aristotle's teaching compared to what they could observe in nature. As noted above, for example, Aristotle had taught that if two balls of the same size were dropped, the heavier of the two would fall faster. This conclusion sounds reasonable. It rings true with our experience and our way of thinking. However, when Galileo tried dropping two such balls from the Leaning Tower of Pisa, they struck the ground at the same time. With experiments like this one, scholars began to see that Aristotle could not necessarily be relied upon. Gradually, the monolith of Aristotelianism crumbled under the weight of empirical evidence.

This questioning of Aristotle was the beginning of what I will call the modern view: *Scientific truth is determined by careful, precise observation in the context of experimentation using the scientific method. There are precise principles that govern the world, and these principles are discernible.*

Notice that there are two parts to this shift in philosophy. The first is the new belief that *observation*, rather than reason, is how we determine truth. The second is a shift from vague generalities to *precise details*. For example, in the experiment with the two balls mentioned above, the question is not only whether one ball hits the ground first. How fast do they fall? Is their speed uniform, or do they accelerate? Can their speed be predicted mathematically to define an underlying principle?

Understanding the motion of falling spheres does not lead immediately to the construction of an air conditioner, but *precise observations form a foundation on which additional observations are made.* Gradually, a body of knowledge is developed, based not on speculation but on precise observation. This body of knowledge then allows predictions for further experimentation. Knowledge in one area allows understanding in seemingly unrelated areas, so that observations about falling spheres on earth allow Isaac Newton to make relevant observations about planetary motion.

It was this new paradigm that led to the explosion of scientific progress that has occurred during the past five hundred years. The apparent "explosion" is actually a large building, constructed one brick at a time.

Note that reason was not abandoned. Reason is necessary to formulate testable hypotheses and to interpret results. However, the fundamental principle is that *reason is inferior to observation*. In other words, if your reason says one thing and the experiment says something else, the experiment is right and you are wrong. Armed with this correction of your original idea, you go back to the drawing board and adjust your hypothesis to come up with another experiment.

Vienna, 1847

Dr. Ignaz Phillip Semmelweis (1818–1865) was excited to be working at a maternity hospital. As he sat down one day to eat in the pub across the street, he could not help but overhear his waitress talking with her friends.

"I want *my* baby delivered by the midwives. My sister is a nurse in the hospital, and she says a lot more of the rich ladies die in the section with the doctors. She says the poor ladies deliver and go home healthy, while a lot of the rich ladies get that purple fever."

"She means puerperal fever," Semmelweis thought, but his parents had taught him that one learns more by listening than by talking, so he kept his mouth shut, discreetly listening to what this woman was saying.

There were two maternity wards, one overseen by midwives, where most of the poorer women delivered, and one overseen by doctors, where the rich women delivered. If what this woman said was true, he needed to figure out why.

After lunch, he went to the head nurses and asked to look at the records in each of the two wards. He was horrified by what he saw. Just as the barmaid had said, there were virtually no cases of puerperal fever in the poor ward, while the rich ward had a high incidence of it. Doctors had more training than midwives, so he had assumed that they did a better job with deliveries. Also, the rich women obviously had access to better food than the poor women. Why would more women die on the rich ward?

(At this point, Semmelweis's view of the world, that doctors provide better care to rich patients than midwives provide to poor patients, was shattered. Instead of persisting in that view, he accepted that his observations meant that his view had to be wrong, and he needed go back to the drawing board to come up with a new theory to explain his observations.)

That evening, Semmelweis dined with his good friend Dr. Jakob Kolletschka. As Jakob's wife brought in the cigars, Phillip told him what he had discovered.

"That is concerning, Phillip," Jakob replied. "I just did an autopsy on one of my patients who died of puerperal fever. I got a nasty nick on my finger in the process. Actually, that finger is getting pretty sore."

Jakob's finger was indeed turning quite red and starting to swell at the site of the cut.

By the next afternoon, Jakob had become quite ill, with a high fever and evidence of shock. When he thought about it, Phillip Semmelweis realized that these symptoms were similar to what happened in puerperal fever. Could there be a connection? Could it be that somehow the fever was transmitted by the transfer of a causative agent between patients? Could Jakob have contracted that same causative agent when he cut his finger?

(Now Semmelweis had a new theory, and he must make additional observations to see whether the theory was worth pursuing.)

Phillip visited the poor ward that afternoon and discreetly observed the midwives. Their delivery technique was not much different from that of the physicians, but there was one huge difference in their conduct. They carefully washed their hands between patients. When asked why, they said they had always done so and just did not like to be dirty. In contrast, doctors, including Semmelweis, had long prided themselves on the amount of blood on their hands, clothing, and laboratory coats.

By the next morning Jakob was dead of his fever. Semmelweis was determined, to honor Jakob's memory, to test his theory. He examined each case of puerperal fever. Usually, he found, the patient who developed the fever had a doctor who had cared for another patient with puerperal fever. The risk of getting the disease was highest when the doctor had recently performed an autopsy on a patient with the fever. Because of this observation and because of the death of his friend, Semmelweis theorized that a "cadaveric factor" was responsible for the condition.

(His additional observations support and clarify his new theory. Now the theory needs to be tested.)

As head of the clinic, he started requiring that the doctors wash their hands before touching the pregnant women. The surgeons were outraged. The very thought that a doctor needed to wash his hands was revolting to them. Semmelweis finally persuaded the surgeons involved at least to try hand washing for two months to see what happened.

(The test was undertaken. The outcomes of patients during the trial period could be compared to the outcomes during the previous two months.)

The results were dramatic. The rate of puerperal fever plummeted, and the incidence of death on the rich wards fell to the lower level seen on the poor wards.

(Semmelweis's theory was validated by the experiment. He gathered additional data over a period of years and then finally informed others in the medical community of his findings.)

Although this discovery had a big impact at his own hospital, when Semmelweis published his findings they were met with great skepticism and even ridicule. The thought that doctors might be *causing* disease was revolting to the medical establishment. Anyway, how on earth did his theories fit into the humoral theory of disease? Semmelweis ultimately suffered a nervous breakdown and wound up in an insane asylum. Ironically, some say, he ultimately died of overwhelming infection in his bloodstream. A few years later, the germ theory of disease was developed and provided a theoretical basis for Semmelweis's discovery.

The findings of Semmelweis were not accepted prior to his death because much of the medical establishment still held to the older view that reason and tradition were the basis for medical treatment. However, Semmelweis demonstrated an early application of the empirical approach to medical treatment (observation is superior to reason and tradition) that would soon dominate medical thought, as it already dominated scientific thought in other areas.

The Result of Empiricism

What is the result of this new paradigm that observation is superior to reason? Without this shift, we would still be at the same level technologically as we were before. Instead, we now enjoy more comfortable and longer lives, because of the painstaking progress made by placing one observation on top of another, abandoning theories that do not

A Christian Perspective

How is truth to be determined from a Christian, biblical perspective? The church supported the Aristotelian view (reason and tradition) for fifteen centuries. Was this biblical? What philosophies were behind the shift to empiricism (the superiority of observation)?

The Problem with Ignorant Reason

According to the Bible, reason alone is a poor way to determine truth. Proverbs warns, "There is a way which seems right to a man, but its end is the way of death" (Prov. 16:25). The period of the judges, for example, was a period of immorality, in which people repeatedly avoided God's direction, and it is summed up with the condemnation "Everyone did what was right in his own eyes" (Judg. 21:25). The decision to do what seemed right, without looking to outside sources, led to moral failure. Repeatedly in scripture, the use of reason in isolation from God is condemned.

Enlightened reason is not condemned but is encouraged. A clear example of this distinction can be found in the book of Job. Job was a wealthy man, with ten children, thousands of livestock, and daily feasts. Then in a single day, all of his children were killed, all of his livestock were killed or taken, and almost all of his servants were killed or taken. In the midst of this suffering, he continued to trust God. Then he developed painful boils all over his body. He must have itched terribly, for he was scraping his skin with a piece of broken pottery while sitting in ashes. His wife and three friends came and sat beside him. Their original intention was to comfort him, but eventually they each began giving him advice. (Perhaps you have friends like that, too.) The first thirty-seven chapters of the book contain Job's thoughts about his sufferings and the thoughts offered by his wife and friends. Many of their thoughts have to do with the nature of the world and the nature of suffering.

Finally, in chapter 38, God speaks: "Who is this that darkens counsel by words without knowledge? Now gird up your loins like a man, and I will ask you, and you instruct Me" (Job 38:2–3). The criticism of their musings is that they were words *without knowledge*. This is analogous to the Aristotelian view, which uses *words*, or more precisely *thoughts*, without any input from outside the mind. The next several chapters contain God's reasoning with Job based on his knowledge of the way things actually are, to help Job gain a proper perspective on life. This is consistent with the modern scientific view, where informed reason is appropriate.

In a biblical view, what is the source of knowledge? Knowledge is obtained by God's revelation. However, in a biblical view, revelation does not come via mystical experiences. There are two sources of revelation cited in scripture. The first is the Bible itself, as articulated in 2 Timothy 3:16–17: "All Scripture is inspired by God and profitable for teaching, for reproof, for correction, for training in righteousness; so that the man of God may be adequate, equipped for every good work." The second source of revelation is God's creation, as Paul discusses in his letter to the Romans: "For since the creation of the world His invisible attributes, His eternal power and divine nature, have been clearly seen, being understood through what has been made" (Rom. 1:20). Therefore, looking at God's creation is an acceptable biblical approach to determining truth. This same approach is also illustrated in Job. As God begins to question him, he often points to the world of nature to help Job understand. For example, he asks, "Who can count the clouds by wisdom . . . ?" (Job 38:37). In other words, you can think all day long, but thought will not tell you how many clouds are in the sky.

The Scientific Revolution Was Due to a Biblical Worldview

Now what, you may ask, do all these Bible verses have to do with the scientific revolution? *Christian individuals and Christian theology of this time period caused the scientific revolution*. This may seem a bold assertion, but it is supported by a great deal of scholarly work and can be illustrated by numerous statements from leaders of science during the centuries of this period of change. Many of the great leaders of the scientific revolution stated explicitly in their writings that they were motivated by a desire to glorify God. They hoped that by their more precise illumination of God's creation, they would inspire men and women to worship him. Nancy Pearcey and Charles Thaxton articulate the facts and controversies surrounding these issues in their book *The Soul of Science: Christian Faith and Natural Philosophy*.[1] I will review only a few of the relevant arguments and provide a few quotes from scientists of the time.

The concept that truth is to be derived from God's revelation in scripture and nature was articulated explicitly by the great scientist Francis Bacon (1561–1626): "Let no one think or maintain that a person can search too far or be too well studied in either the book of God's Word or the book of God's works."[2] Of course "the book of God's Word" refers to the Bible, and "the book of God's works" refers to the entirety of God's creation.

Galileo (1564–1642), whose experiment at Pisa was mentioned above, argued that observation is superior to reason because it would be presumptuous to believe that we know how God thinks; instead, we should go out and look at the world he created.[3] Galileo explicitly criticized the arrogance of those who believed that thought alone could lead to an understanding of such a complex universe. Even if you are an atheist, it does seem the height of human arrogance to believe that with three pounds of brains we could figure out how the universe works without even opening our eyes.

One Christian motivation for scientific endeavor was expressed by the astronomer Johannes Kepler (1571–1630). When asked why he engaged in science, he replied, "To obtain a sample test of the delight of the Divine Creator in His work and to partake of His joy."[4] Robert Boyle, the father of modern chemistry, authored a book titled *Wisdom of God Manifested in the Works of Creation*.[5] In his book *Science and Christianity: Conflict or Coherence*, Henry Schaefer cites many other examples of Christian statements by scientists, not only in Renaissance times but up to the present day.[6]

The view of the typical modern scientist does differ from the view of the typical modern Christian in some ways. The most important difference is that modern science starts out with a presupposition that there is nothing supernatural. In other words, *all* phenomena are explainable based on the natural principles that govern the universe. Divine intervention, which could be defined as God's stepping into the picture and violating natural laws, is assumed not to occur. Of course, Christians as a group would agree that divine intervention is the exception and not the rule. Were it not the exception, it would not be divine *intervention*, and we would be back to Aristotelianism, where nature is unpredictable. The modern Christian, however, would accept the idea that God sometimes heals people supernaturally but would state that supernatural healing is unusual; the modern scientist might not accept supernatural healing as a possibility.

In summary, the individuals responsible for the scientific revolution represented a shift from an Aristotelian view, where truth is determined by reason, to an empiricist view, where truth is determined by observation. In many cases, these luminaries adopted empiricism for Biblical reasons, and pursued science for Christian motivations.

correspond to reality, and adopting new ones by paying careful attention to the world as it actually is.

Difficulties in Medicine

Despite the remarkable advances, progress in medicine lagged far behind progress in other areas of scientific inquiry. In part this delay was due to the need for more knowledge and technology to allow progress in medicine. However, there are three other difficulties in medicine that are not problems in the physical sciences.

Biological Variability

The first difficulty is the individual variability of biological systems. In the incident recounted in chapter 1, as we stood around Julie's stretcher in the emergency room and shocked her heart with 200 joules of electricity, we did not know whether her heart would start beating again or not.

We knew that if we did not shock her, the chances that her heart would start beating again were quite close to zero, even if not exactly zero. We also knew that her chances of survival were much better if we shocked her.

The differences between this and a physics experiment are profound. In physics, if you strike an object with a given amount of force from a given angle, its behavior will be the same every time. Medical treatments, in contrast, are never 100 percent effective, nor are they ever 100 percent ineffective or harmful. Therefore, to assess the effect of a treatment on a disease or condition, it is necessary to treat more than one person and to assess the response *statistically* in comparison to individuals who do not receive the treatment. For example, a given antibiotic may cure 80 percent of cases of bronchitis. If only 5 percent of bronchitis sufferers get better without treatment, this response is excellent. However, it is not like physics, where effects of interventions will be 100 percent.

The Placebo Effect

The second difficulty unique to medical science is the placebo effect. The placebo effect is an apparent benefit that occurs even though a treatment itself has no beneficial physical effects. If I tell one hundred patients that a treatment I administer will help them, many of them will *feel* better whether the treatment actually helps or not. The classic example of this is when patients are given a "sugar pill" rather than a pill containing medicine. Some of the placebo effect is psychological, with the patients feeling better because they expect to feel better, with no physical change in their bodies. Some of the placebo effect may be due to real physical changes that occur from the positive thoughts associated with positive expectations. Some of the placebo effect may be because the symptoms would have improved anyway with no intervention whatsoever.

For example, some people with pneumonia get better even if you bleed them. My grandparents also illustrated this principle for me many years ago.

It is late on a Saturday afternoon in June. I am hot and sweaty, but I don't mind at all. I am six years old, and we have been fishing all day at the little pond my grandparents own in rural Georgia. My parents have cleaned the fish and placed them on ice. Now our 1956 Buick drives up into the dirt driveway of my grandparents' house, only a mile or so from the pond. We go into their living room, which is filled with the aroma of the pecan pie that my grandmother has just baked. In the refrigerator are leftover fried chicken and ham. In the breadbox are biscuits that were first cooked for lunch but are now kept for breakfast the next morning, to be served with hot gravy or cold with the leftover ham.

The living room is fairly dark, with light only from the windows, since these are the days before my grandparents had air conditioning. While I do not mind being hot and sweaty, I do mind sitting quietly in the living room and enduring "grown-up" conversation. I try to sit still, but I become more and more bored.

Inevitably, conversation turns to the arthritic joint pains that afflict both of my grandparents. This is always one of the topics of conversation. Sometimes they say that it is not too bad, and sometimes they report that they are having a lot of pain. Today they report that their symptoms are worse than ever. Finally, I am allowed to go outside to play.

A month later, on our next visit, after another hot day at the pond, I notice that both of my grandparents have new jewelry on their wrists, made of a reddish-brown metal. Although I generally have no interest in jewelry, the sight of my grandfather wearing a bracelet piques my interest.

"What is that?" I ask my grandfather, speaking rather loudly because of his poor hearing.

"This is my new copper bracelet. It's supposed to help arthritis. I got this about three weeks ago, and I feel better than I have in a long time."

Now it is late September. The leaves are changing, and a cool breeze is in the air. We are wearing jackets and picking up pecans under the trees in my grandparents' yard. My grandfather is there with us, and again I notice his bracelet.

"Grandfather, how is your arthritis treating you?"

"Steven, it's a lot worse now. My copper bracelet has quit working. I guess I need another one."

Hopefully, you know more chemistry now than my grandfather did then and recognize that the idea that copper is somehow different after it has been on your wrist for a couple of months is absurd: it is still a copper bracelet. If the old bracelet is not working, a new one will work no better. Hopefully, you realize that wearing a copper bracelet has no effect on arthritis. But if copper bracelets don't help arthritis, why did my grandfather feel better?

Arthritis, by nature, gets better and worse over time, with good days and bad days, good weeks and bad weeks, and good months and bad months. At what stage in this cycle of ups and downs would my grandfather go out and buy a bracelet? People go out of their way to try something new when they have been in a long slump, with prolonged symptoms worse than usual. Whatever my grandfather does, his arthritis will be better a month later: he was in a bad period when he bought it and was bound to go into a better period no matter what. So in this case, the placebo effect was due to the natural history of the disorder, and the copper bracelet, I will assert, had no effect at all.

The Nocebo Effect

A third difficulty in medicine is the converse of the placebo effect. When individuals feel that a treatment will make them worse, they may experience negative reactions that are not caused by the medication. For example, once a patient called me and asked if his cholesterol medication could cause him to get a cold. Usually the symptoms are not so obviously unrelated, but the principle is the same: unpleasant symptoms may occur when the medication is administered that are not caused by the medication. This is called the *nocebo* effect.

Why would someone be such a pessimist? It is not usually pessimism in general but a negative view of medicine. Often a patient will say to me something like "I just can't take medicine." Of course, if this statement is true, they are doomed to live only as long as they would have lived five hundred years ago, since even surgery requires the administration of medicine for pain control. In reality, although we all have different sensitivities to various medications, no one is so different from all others that he is unable to tolerate any medication that other members of his species can tolerate. However, this attitude is a powerful setup for the nocebo effect.

The Double-Blind, Controlled Trial

How does medical science distinguish between the true effects of a treatment and the placebo effect? Part of the approach is to randomly divide a group of people into two groups, one receiving the treatment being tested and the other receiving a fake treatment, with each individual not knowing whether her treatment is the medication or the "sugar pill."

But the other concern is the placebo effect on the doctor. When I give someone a medication, I hope with all my heart that it works. If I am doing the experiment and hoping that my drug is a winner, I will not be objective.

I will want to believe that those receiving the drug have improved. I may think that they look better. I may subtly communicate to the active drug group that they should be better, and to the placebo group that they should not be better, so that their responses to my questions may reflect my expectations. To control for this, drug trials are best when they are "double-blind," meaning that neither the patients nor the doctors know which individual is getting the sugar pill and which is getting the drug. Once the outcomes are recorded and the experiment is complete, everyone can see the results.

As noted earlier, reason alone is a poor tool for determining scientific truth; careful, precise observation is the best method for determining medical facts. For medicine, these determinations are best made in the context of randomized, double-blind controlled trials.

Medicine Catches Up

Because of its particular challenges compared to other sciences, medicine had still not made much progress until the twentieth century. Bloodletting to get the humors in balance, for example, was still widely practiced until the late 1800s. Medical education was still largely an apprenticeship, teaching how things were done, with little emphasis on experimentation and understanding the scientific basis for treatments.

In 1910, a man named Abraham Flexner authored a report on the state of medical education in the United States. Because of this report and its recommendations, medical education caught up with science. In the United States, medical schools changed from a trade-school mentality to a professional-school mentality, training thinkers and leaders who would critically examine new treatments, and play a major role in the development of new science. That was the beginning of the present era of rapid scientific progress in medicine. The result was that during the twentieth century, the average life expectancy increased by thirty years.

Summary

This chapter on philosophy may have been heavy going for you. Before you decide to ignore it and staple these pages together, let me tell you the bottom line: you cannot discover the truth by thinking about it with your eyes closed. To discover the truth, you need to examine the way things actually are with your eyes open. Good ideas are not enough. Cold, hard facts are what we need. This is true in medicine, in science, and in morality. The acceptance of this principle several hundred years ago is the only reason that you can make coffee today without gathering wood and building a fire.

In medicine, we made progress after we learned that the only way to know if a treatment works is to compare it to other treatments. The comparison must be done in such a way that neither the patients nor the doctors know who is getting which treatment. This type of experiment is known as a double-blind, randomized, controlled trial. It eliminates the biases of the participants in order to get at the truth.

In some areas of medicine, biases are harder to eradicate. In chapters 6 and 7, we explore the nature of bias and examine how it affects every aspect of health care.

Notes

1. Nancy Pearcey and Charles Thaxton, *The Soul of Science: Christian Faith and Natural Philosophy* (Wheaton, IL: Crossway, 1994). This book

provides more precise analysis than the loose descriptions of Aristotelianism and modern science I have sketched here. I have chosen to be imprecise to allow for brevity and simplicity. If you wish to study this issue properly, I would encourage you to use Pearcey and Thaxton's book as a starting point.

2. Quoted by Henry F. Schaefer III in *Science and Christianity: Conflict or Coherence?* (Watkinsville, GA: The Apollos Trust, 2003), 15.

3. Pearcey and Thaxton, *Soul of Science*, 34.

4. Schaefer, *Science and Christianity*, 15–16.

5. Ibid., 16–17.

6. Ibid., 7–35.

6

✚

Does Bias Affect Everyone, Even My Doctors and Me?

"So, Dr. Brown," Julie mused, "I shouldn't just accept the good ideas that I read about in these health magazines?"

"That's right, Julie. Even smart people can be wrong. The only way to know if an idea is true is to test it. Good ideas and new therapies must be thoroughly tested in the right kinds of studies before we accept them."

"But what if I feel better? Doesn't that prove that a treatment works? Are you saying that I could experience the placebo effect too?"

"Julie, *all* of us can be affected by the placebo effect, and all of us are affected by bias."

Bias

Have you ever discovered that your memory of an event was different from someone else's? Do you think that you are always the one who is right and the other person is always wrong? Or do you think that maybe you are both right and both wrong?

Bias is the tendency to interpret and remember information in a nonobjective way, usually because of a vested interest in the conclusion. This lack of objectivity is not deliberate. It is completely unconscious, so that when I am biased, I believe that I am completely objective. Stop smiling. The same thing is true for you.

Since bias has the potential to affect every decision, it is important to try to avoid bias in important decisions, like those that affect our health. In this chapter, we will examine how bias affects all of us, and begin to examine how the modern health care system protects us from bias.

An Important Experiment

George Loewenstein and his colleagues conducted a series of experiments that demonstrate just how powerful bias is in our perceptions of reality.[1] These experiments are described in a series of articles that I have listed in note 1. The results were so profound and so surprising that I think it is worthwhile to review their work. To make the experiment easier to understand, I have dramatized it and fabricated details.

It was a cold Saturday morning. Phil would have preferred to sleep in, but the opportunity to participate in a sociology experiment with this kind of compensation was hard to pass up. The advertisement had said that he could receive up to $250 for only three hours of his time. As a graduate student trying to survive on a modest stipend, he really needed the money.

As he and the other volunteers filed in, they were each given a sealed envelope. At 8:30, a professor came into the room and addressed the group. He was wearing a shirt open at the collar, a camelhair blazer, and gray trousers. A pipe protruded from his jacket pocket.

"Ladies and gentleman, we appreciate your willingness to come out on a cold Saturday morning to participate in this project. You are making an important contribution to science today, but I suspect that you are more interested in the contribution science will make to you at the conclusion of the morning." He smiled.

"Each of you has before you a packet of materials. This packet contains documents from an actual lawsuit in another city. In a few minutes, I will ask you to open the packets and begin reading these materials. You will be given two assignments based on your reading and will receive additional compensation that is potentially quite generous, in addition to what you have already been promised, depending on how well you carry out these assignments.

"On December 6, 1972, Gerald Harris, a forty-seven-year-old bank teller, walked into a grocery store owned by Jonathan King. Mr. Harris slipped in a puddle of water and broke his neck. He was out of work for a year but eventually made a full recovery. He sued Mr. King, alleging that his fall was due to King's negligence. He asked for both compensatory damages, to restore his lost wages, and punitive damages, because he felt that King's negligence deserved punishment. After reading the information in the packet, your first assignment is to estimate how much money, if any, was awarded to Mr. Harris at the trial. You will place this estimate in the designated envelope and seal it. The closer you come to the actual amount, the more additional compensation you will receive, up to $100."

At this announcement, there were low whistles and pleased glances around the room.

"Next, you will be paired with another participant. One of you is assigned to the role of Harris, and the other is assigned to the role of King. You are to negotiate with your partner to reach a monetary settlement, each discussing the facts from the point of view to which you have been assigned. On the front of your packet, in addition to your name, is the designation 'Harris' or 'King,' so that you will know as you read which role you will be playing.

"In the negotiation part of the experiment, you will be compensated based on how quickly you reach a settlement. The amount will start at $150, but this amount will decrease as time passes, so that the faster you reach an agreement, the more you will receive in compensation.

"Anyone have any questions? If not, you may begin reading."

Phil looked at the packet. He had been assigned the role of Harris.

"Let's see," he thought, "Harris is the guy who fell."

Phil pulled out the papers and began reading. He started with Harris's testimony at the trial. Harris told the court that he was wearing boots because of the snow outside. Noticing that there were puddles everywhere in the store when he came in, he pointed it out to a manager, who said they were mopping the water up as fast as they could but did not seem to be too concerned. Harris then walked through the produce section. He was being careful but slipped when he stepped on the floor right outside a door marked "employees only." He noted that the floor was especially slippery and quickly learned why. A store employee told him that they had spilled a vat of lard on the floor in the back, and the lard had been tracked out into the main store. The employee was very concerned and sympathetic as they waited for the ambulance. Harris could still move at that point, but he had numbness all over his body from his neck down. Later, when he learned that several employees had tried to get King to move the deep-fat fryer farther from the door, he decided to sue. He could not believe that a store owner would allow a deep-fat fryer containing slippery grease that close to an area where many people walked.

As Phil read the deposition, he was becoming angry at King. It was so irresponsible for him to allow this situation and to neglect those puddles all over the store. He read the rest of the materials, but he remained unconvinced by King's responses. Even though Harris had been involved in previous lawsuits, he felt that the present case was a separate issue. Based on what he had read, he thought that the jury probably awarded Harris at least $500,000.

Across the room from Phil and two rows back, Janice was reading her packet containing exactly the same information. She had been assigned to the role of King. She remembered that he was the guy who owned the store and got sued. Her conclusions from the same information were quite different. December 6, 1972, was the day of the worst snowstorm that town had experienced in one hundred years, and it had been totally unexpected. King had most of his extra employees outside shoveling and salting the snow on the sidewalks to prevent injuries there, with the plan to do more mopping inside a bit later. Consideration had been given to moving the deep-fat fryer, but this was only to bring it closer to the area of the store where fried foods were sold. At that location, it would be close to a door leading out to the store, but a different door to allow efficiency in placing the fried items in the display case. The employee who had spilled the lard had immediately gone to get a sign and ropes to block off the area, but Harris had walked by before the employee could post the sign. Janice also learned from Harris's deposition that he had been involved in two previous lawsuits for injuries that he claimed were the result of negligence.

Janice was disturbed that the store owner had done everything he could to protect his customers in a difficult situation and was now being sued for an unfortunate and unpreventable accident. She knew that juries are often more sympathetic to the injured than to store owners, but she did not see how an honest jury could award Harris anything. She guessed that Harris was awarded nothing.

After everyone had finished placing their guesses in the envelopes, they were conducted to small classrooms for negotiations. Phil and Janice were paired together.

"Could you believe how Harris tried to blame King for his injuries?" Janice asked after they were alone and ready to begin the negotiation process.

"How could he not blame King? King's employee didn't even care that the floor was wet, and King had plenty of chance to move the deep-fat fryer before the accident occurred," Phil responded rather vehemently. He was a little surprised at his emotional reaction to the case, but he felt quite strongly about it.

Despite discussing the case and trying to negotiate, Phil and Janice had still not agreed on a settlement amount when the professor came in to tell them the time was up.

The results were the same all over the building that day. Individuals assigned to the role of King consistently felt that Harris should receive less money. Those assigned to the role of Harris predicted higher awards. The further apart the predictions of a given pair, the less likely they were to reach an agreement. Even though they would get more compensation if they were able to see the other point of view, they could not avoid bias.

The experiment was later repeated, but this time the professor told the participants about the results of the first experiment and warned them that people have a tendency to be biased in favor of the role to which they are assigned. Even so, the results were the same. People continued to favor the party whose identity they assumed. When asked how the information about potential bias helped them, the participants reported that it helped them understand how the *other person* might be biased, but they denied that they themselves were biased.

Do you get the point? We all think that bias is something that happens to *other people*, when it is actually something that happens to us, too. Some years ago, a survey was done among medical residents about the effects that gifts from pharmaceutical sales representatives might have on medical practice. While 61 percent of the residents felt that gifts did not affect their practice, 84 percent believed that gifts affected the practice of other physicians.[2]

I am happy to concede that bias occurs among doctors. I also want you to realize that it happens to butchers, bakers, candlestick makers, and the members of whatever occupation you practice.

The implications are profound and universal. The placebo effect is a manifestation of bias, so that *I cannot tell for myself* if a treatment I receive is working, even if I seem to feel a lot better or a lot worse. For the same reason, I cannot rely on the testimonials of others to determine whether a treatment is effective for them. To know if a treatment works, we need a double-blind, randomized, controlled trial, as discussed in chapter 5.

Personal Applications

The concept of bias has personal, practical applications, apart from their relevance to science and health care. An obvious example is how our lack of objectivity about our own experience plays a major role in our understanding of

A Christian Perspective

The potential for self-deception illustrated by the placebo effect is also articulated in scripture. Jeremiah tells us, "The heart is more deceitful than all else and is desperately sick; who can understand it?" (Jer. 17:9). This warning should keep us from simply relying on our own thoughts or feelings to determine truth.

This potential for self-deception is an additional reason that we cannot make ethical decisions by reason alone. When we try to reason out what is right and wrong with no outside input, our lack of objectivity makes it impossible to do so accurately. The relativism of today, with its rejection of any absolute standard of right and wrong, leads inevitably to the abuses of power that have been seen in the corporate world and the political world. We need an outside standard of right and wrong and must be vigilant in measuring ourselves against it.

ourselves and others. Remember the episode in the 1960s sitcom *Gilligan's Island* where this lack of objectivity is acted out? An event that occurred in the lives of the seven people stranded on the tropical island is presented from each person's viewpoint. Inevitably, each person remembers the event with himself or herself as the hero and everyone else demonstrating selfishness, foolishness, and cowardice. I suspect you can remember a time when you had a conflict with someone, and in discussing how the conflict came about, you have realized that the other person's recollection or understanding of the event is entirely different from your own. Who is right? Do you not think that the other person might be at least partly right?

I must be very careful to listen to the viewpoints of those around me if I am to have any hope of understanding the truth about myself. I must also be vigilant to avoid bias in making wise decisions for those for whom I am responsible. I must interpret the information I receive from others in the context of their biases, whether they are physicians or salespeople or friends. Most important in the health-care system, I must understand the effects that bias has on those responsible for my health care.

How Does Modern Medicine Try to Protect Us against Bias?

Modern science recognizes the problem of bias, and there are many protections in place in modern medicine to avoid the effects of bias. As an example, let us consider how drugs are developed.

Typically, a drug starts out as an idea. Someone comes to believe, based on theoretical considerations or chance observations, that a substance may be helpful in treating a disease. They then must convince someone to pay for research to determine if this is so. That "someone" may be the head of their department at the pharmaceutical company, or it may be a committee at the National Institutes of Health that reviews their proposal for a research grant.

After extensive testing in the laboratory and in animals, if the evidence suggests that the substance may indeed be helpful, application is made to the Food and Drug Administration (FDA) to allow testing of the substance in humans. A committee of people who are not supposed to have any vested interest in the decision reviews the data and decides whether to allow the product to be tested in humans or to direct that further testing be done with animals.

How is the testing done in humans? It is done in the context of a prospective, double-blind, randomized, controlled trial, as discussed in chapter 5. Each individual is evaluated to see what their response has been by doctors who do not know whether they received the actual drug or a placebo. The researchers faithfully record whatever they are told by the patients. Laboratory and x-ray results on each subject are reviewed and analyzed. The results are scrutinized not only for improvement in the underlying disease but also for any adverse effects of treatment. While a positive response to treatment is likely to be common, adverse effects are often uncommon, perhaps afflicting only one in a hundred or one in a thousand recipients of a new drug.

After the results of the trial are analyzed by the investigators, if they feel that product has merit, they present these results to the FDA. Another committee whose members are supposed to have no vested interest in the outcome then decides whether the product should be approved for general usage, and if so, under what conditions.

If a product is approved, the FDA continues to provide what is called *after-marketing surveillance*. If I prescribe a medication to you and you come back and tell me that your hair fell out, I am not supposed to decide if it happened because of the medication. I am simply supposed to report it to the FDA. Even if I don't think that the product had anything to do with your hair loss, if the FDA receives five reports from Texas and twenty from California and three from Georgia, the possibility that hair loss may be an adverse effect has to be taken seriously. Of course, the same process is followed with more serious adverse effects, such as death or kidney failure.

At each step of the process, then, protections are in place to prevent bias from misleading us. The system is not perfect, but it attempts to provide appropriate protections.

Similar protections are present in the world of research. If I as a researcher observe something that I think is important, I record the relevant observations in a paper and submit it to a medical journal for publication. The editor sends my paper to two other researchers who are experts in my field. Those investigators review my work, and each sends a review to the editor. They may recommend that the paper be published as written, but typically they recommend that additional, confirmatory experiments be done prior to publication. This process is called *peer review*, and medical publications that use this process are sometimes referred to as *peer-reviewed journals*.

As an individual in practice, I also have some protection against bias. Groups of experts develop and publish guidelines for the diagnosis and treatment of certain conditions. Since every patient is different, there often remains a level of subjectivity, but guidelines help to ensure proper care by creating a consensus about what approaches are best. In areas where guidelines do not exist, the medical literature is based on double-blind placebo controlled trials, so that if I study the literature, I at least have objective information to guide my decisions.

Summary

Bias is part of the human condition. Even when I believe that I am objective, my emotions, my beliefs, and my vested interests affect my judgment. As a doctor, I must do all I can to protect my patients from bias. As a patient, you must do all you can to protect yourself from bias.

The world of medicine has developed institutional and governmental protections against bias. Despite these protections, as we will see in the next chapter, a lack of recognition of bias has resulted in departures of modern medicine from true science and from a Christian worldview. Understanding bias can help you avoid a lot of traps in the medical maze.

Notes

1. I was introduced to these experiments in a wonderful article by J. Dana and G. Loewenstein, "A Social Science Perspective on Gifts to Physicians from Industry," *New England Journal of Medicine* 290 (2003): 252–55. This article summarizes the experiments. The original articles referred to in this paper are listed below:

G. Loewenstein, S. Issacharoff, C. Camerer, and L. Babcock, "Self-Serving Assessments of Fairness and Pretrial Bargaining," *Journal of Legal Studies* 12 (1992): 135–59.

L. Babcock, G. Loewenstein, S. Issacharoff, and C. Camerer, "Biased Judgments of Fairness in Bargaining," *American Economic Review* 85 (1995): 1337–42.

L. Babcock, X. Wang, and G. Loewenstein, "Choosing the Wrong Pond: Social Comparisons That Reflect a Self-Serving Bias," *Quarterly Journal of Economics* 111 (1996): 1–19.

L. Babcock and G. Loewenstein, "Explaining Bargaining Impasse: The Role of Self-Serving Biases," *Journal of Economic Perspectives: A Journal of the American Economic Association* 11 (1997): 109–26.

L. Babcock, G. Loewenstein, and S. Issacharoff, "Creating Convergence: Debiasing Biased Litigants," *Law and Social Inquiry* 22 (1997): 401–13.

2. This observation was cited by Dana and Loewenstein, "Social Science," with their original reference being M. Steinman, M. Shilpak, and S. McPhee, "Of Principles and Pens: Attitudes of Medicine Housestaff toward Pharmaceutical Industry Promotions," *American Journal of Medicine* 110 (2001): 551–57.

7

✚

Avoiding the Traps
That Bias Sets for You

"Dr. Brown," Julie said thoughtfully, "I guess you've convinced me that I can be biased. I can see that doctors can be biased too. How often does bias affect your decisions?"

An Example from the World of Appliances

"The washing machine quit working today."

We called a company that had repaired other appliances for us. A repairman whom we had not seen before answered the call.

He was about five and a half feet tall and looked trim and athletic. He wore new overalls, with the edge of a T-shirt visible around his neck, partially covered by a crisp red bandanna. He smelled more of cologne than of the grease that you would expect given his occupation.

After spending a half hour alone with our washer, he climbed up from the basement to tell us the bad news. At least it was bad news for *us*.

"The washer needs a new motor. That would cost you $200. I happen to sell used washers on the side, and I could sell you one that I've reconditioned for $225. That would be almost as good as getting a new one. I guarantee the ones I've reconditioned for ninety days."

What's wrong with this picture? If the repairman fixes my washer, he gets whatever his employer pays him per hour. If he claims that it can't be fixed and succeeds in selling me one he's reconditioned, he gets whatever his employer pays him per hour, plus $225. He then hauls off my old washer, fixes it, and sells it to someone else for $225. No wonder he was better dressed than the average repairman. I decided to get a second opinion.

Unfortunately, just like the world of appliance repair, medicine does not always succeed in protecting us from conflicts of interest. Bias is everywhere and sneaks in through every crack in the best-designed wall. Understanding bias, however, allows us to develop strategies to minimize its effects.

In this chapter, we will first consider how bias affects doctors. Next, we will examine how bias affects pharmaceutical companies. We will then look at how ethical principles and institutional and governmental regulations try to protect us from bias. Finally, I will present some practical applications.

How Does Bias Affect Doctors?

Every time we interact with a doctor, or any other individual, each person has incentives to behave in a certain way. If we understand those incentives, we will at least understand how others are likely to behave in a questionable situation. For example, in a typical *fee for service* system of reimbursement, doctors are paid for what they do and are paid more for doing more. A surgeon typically makes most of her money by doing surgery. Therefore, in a borderline case, she has an incentive to recommend surgery. If she knows that and she is honest, she will try to be very careful to avoid letting that bias influence her and will seek to use objective criteria to make her decision.

A patient of mine went to a surgeon because of high calcium levels. One treatment for this condition is surgery to remove the parathyroid glands. After completing his evaluation, the surgeon said to her, "I love to operate, but I don't think that an operation is the right thing for you, at least at this point." The surgeon recognized and articulated his bias, and he avoided allowing his bias let him make the wrong decision.

I have not been able to find this documented (maybe it's an urban legend), but I was told in medical school that in the early days of health maintenance organizations (HMOs), one company decided to require preapproval for hysterectomies. In other words, before a doctor could perform a hysterectomy on a patient, she had to call the insurance company and ask them to approve the procedure. They did not tell the doctors, but the company's policy was that preapproval would be granted automatically to every doctor who requested it, no matter what reason the doctor gave for the surgery. Disturbingly, the rate of hysterectomies fell by 50 percent. Probably some of those doctors had been deliberately doing unnecessary surgery. However, I suspect that most had justified the procedures in their own minds, convincing themselves and their patients that they were necessary. But when required to explain the rationale to someone else, they knew that their reasoning would not withstand scrutiny.

Because of this systematic bias, payers have experimented with alternative forms of physician reimbursement. Some HMOs have given primary care physicians a budget for each patient, with money from that budget being used to pay for tests and referrals to specialists and money left over going into the pocket of the primary care physician. This creates a bias *against* tests and referrals. The latest approach in the payment of doctors has been "capitation," where the doctor is paid a certain number of dollars for each person covered in the plan. Since the doctor is paid whether he does anything or not, he has an incentive to do as little as possible.

No matter what form of reimbursement you choose, there will be a conflict of interest. You can choose in which direction the conflict lies and control its magnitude, but you cannot eliminate it.

When I was offered my first contract to start in private practice, I hired an attorney to review it. Most of what he told me was of little lasting value. However, he gave me one critical piece of advice I have never forgotten. He told me that *the most important part of any contract is the people who sign it*. If the people entering into an agreement are honorable and honest, they will try to treat each other properly no matter what is in the contract. If they are dishonorable and dishonest, they will try to cheat each other no matter what is written in the contract.

And so it is with the practice of medicine. If your doctor is honorable, he will try to treat you properly. If your insurance company is honorable, it will try to treat you honorably. If your doctor or insurance company is dishonorable, you need to do all you can with checks, balances, and government regulation to protect your health.

As discussed in chapter 3, my training as a doctor teaches me to make decisions for patients based on the patient's interests, regardless of what it costs me personally. To the extent that the training works, and for as long as it works, that process affords some protection to my patients. In addition, doctors who care about their reputation in the medical community, a community that values honesty and conservatism, also have a vested interest in "doing the right thing" regardless of financial incentives to the contrary.

New Screening Tests and Direct-to-Consumer Advertising

One of the newest problems in medicine is the development of expensive screening tests that can make a lot of money for doctors. The proper approach to proving that these tests are useful would be double-blind randomized controlled trials. If a test demonstrates benefits in this context, the medical community will adopt it en masse, and insurance companies will end up paying for it. The new alternative approach is to market a test directly to the public, claiming (without proper evidence) that it has value in detecting problems. At the same time, advertising and sales representatives market the test to doctors as a tool to make money. In our affluent, consumer-oriented economy, there are a lot of people who like the idea of paying five hundred dollars for a new, high-tech test that is not covered by insurance and therefore not available to the general public. Let's look at an example.

Electron Beam CT Scanning

In 1996, I was attending a conference in St. Louis about controlling cholesterol. At the buffet breakfast, I overheard an open conversation behind me about "this new machine that is making us all kinds of money." I turned around and joined others in listening to a cardiologist discuss his new electron beam CT scanner (EBCT). This device detects calcium in the coronary arteries, the vessels that provide blood to the heart. Shortly before I overheard this conversation, these machines had been marketed throughout the country as a way to detect coronary disease earlier than other tests could do it. It was known that coronary calcification is sometimes associated with significant narrowing in the arteries to the heart. However, there were no good data defining how often this association occurred or whether such information would be useful.

When EBCT machines became available, promoters invited journalists to undergo free scans. This resulted in favorable reports in popular magazines, newspapers, and television shows. The test was not covered by insurance, since it had no established value as a medical test. Ironically, the lack of coverage increased its popularity among people who could afford five hundred bucks for a medical test. The cardiologist at the conference was talking about how his patients were clamoring for this test and how when calcium was found in their arteries, the pictures were so vivid that the patients became very motivated to get their risk factors under control.

So what is wrong with a test like this? Is it not best to get as much information as possible? To answer these questions, I need to educate you about some of the limitations of medical testing.

Limitations of Medical Tests

No medical test is perfect. For example, EBCT does not actually detect blockages; it only detects calcium. The test results can be normal, and you may still have severe blockages. The test results can be markedly abnormal, and you may still have no blockages at all. Such imperfection is a characteristic of all medical tests. To know whether a test is useful or useless, you must know *how often* the test is misleading and how often it is correct. With a new test, you cannot know until you try it out on a good many people and study the results. You also must compare the information provided by the test with information that could be obtained in other ways. In 1990, there was not enough information to know whether EBCT helped or not. As of 2002, we knew that the predictive value of the test was the same as simply asking the patient her age, her family history, her blood pressure, and her cholesterol level.

The second question that must be answered about a test is what should be done with the information it provides. In the case of this test, in 1996 and even now, no useful information is obtained with EBCT, since no one knows how the information obtained should change therapy. If your blood pressure is high, we know how to treat it. If EBCT predicts blockages, we do not know whether we help you by doing more tests or changing your medications or not.

Wouldn't doing more tests always be useful? Let's consider the example of mammography. Since mammography became available, doctors have debated at what age women should begin having mammograms. At present, the American Cancer Society recommends that women begin having mammography at age forty. Let's suppose that, instead, mammography is done on twenty-year-old women. Women of this age are unlikely to have breast cancer, even if they have an abnormal mammogram. Of course, the mammograms of most twenty-year-old women will be normal. Let us suppose for the sake of argument that out of 100 abnormal mammograms in twenty-year-old women, 99 of these women will not have breast cancer and one will have breast cancer. Let us further suppose that you would have to do 10,000 mammograms on twenty-year-old women to find 100 that are abnormal. Now, each abnormal mammogram will lead to further testing, which might include an immediate breast biopsy or follow-up mammography in three months.

To locate one breast cancer, perhaps 99 women face the risks associated with a breast biopsy, including a small risk of death from anesthesia. All of the 100 women with abnormal mammograms experience the anguish of fear that they may have breast cancer and the torture of waiting two weeks for the biopsy results. The other question, of course, is whether you even helped the one woman in whom you found breast cancer. If her cancer would have been discovered in some other way, such as feeling a lump, then you have not helped her by doing a mammogram. If the early diagnosis does not change her outcome, such as it would if the cancer has already spread, or if the cancer would still have been diagnosed in time without the mammogram, then 10,000 women have been through a mammogram, and 100 have had an operation, for absolutely nothing. Of course, since the test is not perfect, there may be another woman in those 10,000 who has breast cancer not seen on the mammogram, and she may delay evaluation of the lump that she finds, believing that it cannot be cancer since her mammogram was normal.

It is because of concerns like this that mammography is not recommended until women are older and therefore at higher risk of breast cancer. In an older woman, an abnormal mammogram is more likely to be caused by breast cancer, so that a smaller number of healthy women will suffer emotionally and physically in order to diagnose one true case of breast cancer.

It is important to understand, however, that these same concerns apply to all types of medical screening tests. How do we know what approach is correct? How do we know when a test is helpful and in what group of people? You guessed it: by prospective, double-blind, randomized controlled trials.

There was a time when it was considered appropriate to do chest x-rays as a screening test in adult smokers to try to find early lung cancers. It was subsequently found that this accomplished nothing, since even when it did lead to earlier diagnosis, there was no change in outcome—the cancers diagnosed earlier had already spread. The only difference was that the individuals so afflicted spent more of their last days knowing that they had cancer. Testing for prostate cancer with a blood test has also undergone similar changes in recent years with the realization that many elderly men with elevated levels of prostate-specific antigen die of causes other than prostate cancer, whether or not they go through the risks and side effects of prostate surgery, radiation, or medical therapy for cancer. For any medical test to be appropriate, it is imperative to understand its limitations and to determine whether the knowledge gained is helpful or harmful to the patient.

Dubious Tests

In the case of electron beam CT scanning, results can be "normal" for people with coronary artery disease and "abnormal" for people without coronary disease. In addition, at the time of this writing, fully ten years after the conversation I overheard, we still do not know what to do with the information gained through the test. If a young person's test results are abnormal, do they deserve more aggressive treatment of cholesterol? Should they undergo stress testing or coronary angiography? If the test is normal, should they be treated less aggressively?

On Valentine's Day 2002, a paper was published in the *New England Journal of Medicine* about electron beam CT scanning. It concluded:

> Finally, we must recognize that at least some informed members of the public will realize that a major reason for providing these unnecessary tests is that physicians profit from them. In fact, many might conclude, quite reasonably, that remuneration is the key factor. This kind of suspicion harms the profession itself and the perception of its commitment to patients. Therefore, a good case can be made that professional ethics prohibits providing unproven diagnostic screening tests, even if there is substantial demand from patients. Rather, physicians should be instructing patients that such tests are unnecessary and using their energy for the appropriate development of evidence regarding the efficacy of these tests.[1]

I suspected that there would be many letters to the editor complaining about this article. Instead, there was only one. All three of the individuals who authored it had financial interests in electron beam CT scanners.[2]

Electron beam CT scanning is only one example of a number of tests and procedures being promoted directly to the public without the benefit of scientific evidence. It is a sad state of affairs when, in the interest of profit, new technologies are deprived of appropriate evaluation. If patients are able to get these tests by writing a check, it is difficult to enroll them in prospective double-blind, randomized, controlled trials to determine if they afford real benefit. The general public is deprived of potential medical advances, and the wealthy public is hoodwinked into receiving tests of no value.

Of course, one predictable result of abnormal test results is that they lead to more tests and procedures. Just as the unfortunate women with abnormal mammograms but no breast cancer undergo breast biopsies, the men and women with abnormal EBCT scans go on to receive stress testing, angiography, and other cardiac tests. This result, the performance of additional medical tests, has not missed the attention of those who promote these screening tests. The five hundred dollars paid by the individual is only the beginning. After the test is found to be abnormal, the individual is given a diagnosis of coronary artery disease, and the testing that is reimbursed by insurance or governmental payers begins. This result is readily exploited in older patients, in whom calcification, which is all the test really detects, is part of the normal aging process.

In his book *Should I Be Tested for Cancer?* Dr. H. Gilbert Welch explores in detail the issues surrounding various screening tests and explains why more is not always better.[3] When a doctor recommends a test, ask why the test is right for you. Has it been validated in people like you? What is the evidence that it will prevent a bad health outcome? Is it a new test or one that has stood the test of time? What are the alternatives? What does a normal result mean? What does an abnormal result mean? How accurate is the test? What will we do differently if the test results are abnormal?

The Biggest Challenge for the Doctor

Few doctors will try to sell you unproven screening tests. Not many doctors will do unnecessary surgery. However, all of us doctors at one time or another will settle for *mediocrity*. This too is an issue of bias, because no one sets out to be mediocre. We just tell ourselves that we are doing our best, when instead we are cutting corners. Although mediocrity is so common it can be hard to recognize, it is not hard to recognize thoroughness and excellence when you see them, because they stand out in contrast to mediocrity.

The pressures of everyday practice can crush the ideals of even the most devoted doctors. Since doctors are paid based on how many patients they see, the system teaches that quantity is more important than quality. With overhead rising and reimbursement falling, doctors are under pressure to see more patients just to maintain the same income. Everyone therefore pays another price: the doctor is in a hurry and does not listen, the patient is frustrated, and medical mistakes are more likely.

Most of the frustration with modern medicine is not a reaction to incompetence or dishonesty; instead, it is a reaction to a lack of attentive listening, compassionate understanding, and personalized direction. Doctors who provide the best care pay the price of longer hours and smaller paychecks. My goal as a physician is to maintain that type of commitment to the welfare of my patients, despite pressures to the contrary. Your goal as a patient is to find a doctor with that type of commitment. Unfortunately, it is getting harder to do so.

The Marine Corps motto is *semper fidelis*: always faithful. This motto captures the concept of a rock-solid commitment to a standard of perfection. This same motto should characterize your doctor when it comes to your medical care. That means listening to what you have to say long enough to understand your problem. It means asking you enough questions to obtain relevant information, information that you probably don't even think is relevant. It means examining you carefully. It means not jumping to conclusions before considering all the possibilities. It means keeping up with the latest medical breakthroughs. It means carefully applying the best treatment and patiently trying alternatives if the first treatment does not work. It means taking the time to explain and to answer your questions. Obviously, perfection is not a standard that any doctor will meet all the time. But if your doctor does not even *aspire* to perfection, find another doctor.

Dr. Michael Roizen and Dr. Mehmet Oz wrote a very helpful book entitled *You: The Smart Patient*.[4] Some of the suggestions that these authors make relate to encouraging thoroughness by your doctor. For example, they suggest assembling your health history in a form that will help your doctor obtain the information that he needs quickly. They also suggest that while you are in the hospital, you keep a box of disposable hand wipes at your bedside to encourage doctors, nurses, and visitors to cleanse their hands before they make contact with you to help avoid infection. Their suggestions demonstrate an understanding of human frailty, including the frailty of health-care providers. I am embarrassed that my profession needs this kind of encouragement to do what we ought to do anyway, but realistically, the more encouragement anyone has, the easier it is to demonstrate excellence.

One manifestation of mediocrity may be allowing you to make your own medical decisions with minimal input or contradiction from the doctor. If you tell your doctor that you want to take garlic pills instead of the prescription medication that she recommended to treat your high cholesterol, and she just says, "OK," you need to find another doctor. *The doctor's job is not to make you happy but to keep you healthy.* There is nothing easier for the doctor than to acquiesce to your demands for antibiotics that you don't need or to agree to whatever alternative therapy is in the latest magazine. A good doctor tries to decide what treatment is best for you based on her more extensive knowledge and skill. She will explain why the treatment she has recommended is superior, or she will discuss the pros and cons of the alternative you suggest if it is a viable alternative. Your wishes as the patient are important, but they should not be the doctor's only consideration in formulating a plan. The same principle applies if you are worried about the risks of a test or a procedure. The doctor should explain the reasons for a test or operation and address your concerns. If you need the test, you need it, and simply letting your questions result in its cancellation is not good medical care. You have the right to make your own decisions, but the doctor has the responsibility to provide you with complete information.

The Pharmaceutical Industry's Bias

Sometimes the pharmaceutical industry makes bad decisions due to bias. According to published reports, the story of Vioxx illustrates how bias can mislead even those with a strong vested interest in seeing things accurately. At this point, it is not clear how much harm Vioxx does or in what populations it may do harm. Nonetheless, the history of this drug demonstrates how bias affects how we view things. In other cases, the industry makes choices that are based on bad ethics from the beginning. The reports about Natrecor illustrate this problem and will be recounted after I summarize the Vioxx debacle.

Vioxx: Bad Decisions with Good Intentions

In May 1999, Vioxx was first marketed in the United States for the treatment of arthritis pain. Older drugs to treat arthritis pain, with the exception of Tylenol, all had a substantial risk of causing ulcers. Doctors and patients were now delighted to have a new arthritis pill without such a high risk of stomach problems. Sales went through the roof.

On November 23, 2000, a study was published looking at the differences between Vioxx and the older drug naproxen. It confirmed that the incidence of stomach problems was lower with Vioxx but also showed the surprising result that the incidence of heart attacks in the group on Vioxx was four times higher than in the group on naproxen.[5]

The increased incidence of heart attacks was ascribed to a beneficial effect of naproxen, however, rather than to a harmful effect of Vioxx. Aspirin has long been used for cardiac protection, because it interferes with the clots that cause heart attacks and strokes. It was known that naproxen also could interfere with clot formation. Prior to this study, those taking Vioxx had been discouraged from taking aspirin for cardiac protection due to a fear that Vioxx might still cause stomach ulcers. After this study, scientists felt that patients taking Vioxx should be encouraged to resume their aspirin. It was hoped that this would solve the problem.[6]

On February 7, 2001, there was a meeting between the FDA and Merck, the company that manufactured Vioxx.[7] The FDA was concerned that perhaps naproxen was not beneficial and that instead Vioxx might be harmful. The Arthritis Drugs Advisory Committee of the FDA voted unanimously that physicians should be made aware of the possibility that Vioxx might increase the risk of heart attack.

The next day, Merck notified its three thousand sales representatives that they should not initiate discussions about the FDA advisory meeting. If a physician asked about the study showing an increased risk of heart attack, they were only to point out that the study showed a decreased risk of stomach problems and then indicate that they could not discuss the study further. Merck's marketing department developed materials that claimed that Vioxx was associated with fewer cardiac deaths than other arthritis medicines. These materials were based on older studies that involved only low-dose, short-term use of Vioxx. In other words, according to Henry Waxman, U.S. representative from California, Merck deliberately chose to suppress the notion that its drug might cause heart attacks.[8] Of course, this decision was consistent with Merck executives' own interpretation of the data: Vioxx did not cause problems with the heart, and the difference between the two groups in the study was due to the protective effects of naproxen.

In September 2004, three and a half years later, a new trial showed that patients taking Vioxx for more than eighteen months had a higher risk of heart attack than those not on Vioxx, and as a result, Merck voluntarily removed Vioxx from the market.[9] In the group of patients on Vioxx, 1.5 percent per year had a "serious thrombotic event" (including things like stroke and heart attack), compared with 0.78 percent per year in the placebo group. The study had been done not to assess the cardiac effects of Vioxx but instead to determine whether Vioxx prevents colon cancer.[10]

The reaction to the removal of Vioxx from the market was intriguing. When Vioxx was promptly removed from the market after the new trial data became available in 2004, the *Lancet* published an editorial praising Merck for its rapid action in light of this new information.[11] As more information became public about Merck's decision to take a strong position against the concerns raised by the study comparing Vioxx to naproxen in 2000, the *Lancet* changed its position and published an editorial critical of Merck and the FDA. They concluded that Merck and the

FDA "acted out of ruthless, short-sighted, and irresponsible self-interest."[12]

Joseph Alpert, a professor of medicine at the University of Arizona, was more sympathetic. Alpert had been one of the many individuals outside Merck who reviewed the information available in 2002 and concluded at the time that the addition of aspirin to Vioxx was a reasonable approach. Like others, inside and outside Merck, he had felt that this would protect the patients from any potential harm and allow them to experience the benefits provided by Vioxx. In an editorial published in the *American Journal of Medicine*, he pointed out:

> Every Merck employee is well aware of the potential for staggering lawsuits if a drug is launched, and it causes myocardial infarcts [heart attacks] and CVAs [strokes]. Merck as a corporation may be severely damaged if not destroyed by the liability involved in the Vioxx debacle. If Merck executives knew about the cardiovascular risks and suppressed them, they also knew that they might be accused of felony once such information came to light. No one in these circumstances would take such a risk.[13]

While Merck had a vested interest in the success of Vioxx, it also had a powerful vested interest in recognizing and dealing with any potential problems with Vioxx rather than sweeping them under the rug. To put this matter into context, Merck has always been a responsible corporate citizen, supporting products important to the public health that are not very profitable, such as vaccines.[14]

At this point, faithful reader, let's apply what we have learned about bias in earlier chapters. We know that all of us are subject to bias. Therefore, we know that the executives at Merck were subject to bias. As hard as they might try, they will not be entirely objective in evaluating negative information about a very profitable drug. Therefore, it is quite possible, and even probable, that in 2002 they sincerely believed that Vioxx did not cause heart attacks. As Alpert points out, their interests, in reality, would have been better protected if they had publicized the FDA recommendations.

Selling to Greed: Bad Decisions with Bad Intentions

In 2001, a new drug called Natrecor was approved by the FDA for the treatment of congestive heart failure in patients who were sick enough to be admitted to the hospital.[15] The basis for the approval was that when compared with nitroglycerin, patients felt a little better and had better pressure readings on invasive testing with Natrecor. There was no difference in death or the need for repeat hospitalization. Of course, this is a very weak justification for approval of a new, expensive drug. (Natrecor costs about fifty times as much as nitroglycerin.) Indeed, this drug was never approved for use by the European Agency for the Evaluation of Medicinal Products (the European equivalent of the FDA). The original studies of the drug also raised concerns about a possible increased risk of death. This concern was supported by reports released in 2005 showing increased risk of both death and kidney failure.[16] To summarize, the drug was approved by the FDA based on weak studies looking at small improvements in how patients felt, and the only approved use of the drug was for patients who had congestive heart failure bad enough to require hospitalization.

According to Dr. Eric Topol, chairman of cardiovascular medicine at the Cleveland Clinic, the company that manufactures Natrecor began encouraging physicians to use it for outpatients, giving them an infusion once a week as a "tune-up." There was never any evidence that this would be of significant benefit to the patients, but the sales representatives were encouraged to provide doctors with information on how much money they could make when billing Medicare for this service. The result was that in 2005, ten times as much of the drug was used in outpatients as in inpatients, with projected sales in 2005 of $700 million.[17] Of course, with the new data on the increased risk of death and renal failure, the widespread use of this drug for an unproved indication was revealed to be even more than a waste of money: it might be physically abusive. With this new information, sales of Natrecor have plummeted again. Studies are now underway to determine whether the apparent increased risk of death and kidney failure are real.

You may remember the old saying that "you can't cheat an honest man." The saying refers to the fact that most swindling schemes play on the greed of the person being cheated. Any doctor should be suspicious when someone tries to sell him a product based on how much money it can make for him, rather than based on what it can do to help his patients.

In this example, salespeople from a drug company were *openly* appealing to the greed of physicians. I am embarrassed to admit this, because the fact that salespeople take this approach implies that some doctors respond to it. Doctors like this are selling the lives of their patients and violating standards of professionalism. Companies that encourage this sort of conduct by doctors are shirking their responsibility to the health-care consumer.

When a doctor recommends a treatment, ask why it is right for you. Has it been tested in people like you? What is the evidence that it will prevent a bad health outcome? Is it a new treatment, or one that has stood the test of time? What are the alternatives?

An Ethics Approach to Avoiding Bias

Consider again that unconscious bias allows us to do things that are wrong and convince ourselves that we are right. One of the central tenets of Judeo-Christian ethics attacks bias by calling us to put ourselves in the other person's shoes. In Matthew 7:12, Jesus says, "In everything, therefore, treat people the same way you want them to treat you, for this is the Law and the Prophets."

Notice that the Golden Rule does not say, "Do to others what you think is right." Instead, it encourages us to get outside our own viewpoint, to put ourselves in the other person's shoes and treat them the way we would want to be treated if we were in their position. The Golden Rule combats bias by encouraging thought from the viewpoint of others.

The Golden Rule exists in some form in many of the world's religions, including Hinduism, Buddhism, Judaism, Confucianism, and Islam. In some cases, it is restricted to "brothers" or coreligionists. In many cases, it is stated negatively, admonishing the adherent *not* to do things to others that they would not want done to themselves. But with these qualifications, the principle is essentially universal.[18]

John F. Kennedy invoked this universal principle to fight one of the most insidious forms of bias: racism. In 1963, he ordered National Guardsmen to protect two black students as they enrolled at the University of Alabama. In an address to the American people that night, he stated:

> The heart of the question is whether all Americans are to be afforded equal rights and equal opportunities, whether we are going to treat our fellow Americans as we want to be treated. If an American, because his skin is dark, cannot eat lunch in a restaurant open to the public, if he cannot

send his children to the best public school available, if he cannot vote for the public officials who will represent him, if, in short, he cannot enjoy the full and free life which all of us want, then who among us would be content to have the color of his skin changed and stand in his place? Who among us would then be content with the counsels of patience and delay?[19]

Kennedy not only *verbally* invoked the Golden Rule; he *metaphorically* invoked it by inviting prejudiced and insensitive white Americans imaginatively to change their skin color and then listen to their "counsels of patience and delay." A little more than a hundred years earlier, Abraham Lincoln invoked the same principle against racism when he said, "As I would not be a slave, so I would not be a master."[20]

This principle also means being willing to ask whether an action even *looks* unethical to that other person. I remember hearing a speaker once remark, "The reason that most people feel guilty is that they are guilty." In the same way, if an action looks unethical, there is a good chance that it *is* unethical. Just imagine your enemies watching you all the time and being able to broadcast your behavior on CNN. Such self-examination is good for those who depend on you.

How do we apply this to health care? When a doctor talks about the options for your treatment, ask what she would want if she were the patient.

Governmental and Institutional Regulation to Avoid Bias

All the problems discussed in this chapter have occurred despite heavy regulation of the health-care industry. Can you imagine what would happen without such regulation?

(Hold that thought. You'll find out the answer in part 3.) Doctors are licensed and regulated by the states. In addition, some standards of qualification and practice are upheld by insurers, including the federal government via Medicare.

Drugs are released for sale only after evaluation for safety and efficacy by the FDA. As we saw above, even though the system usually works, it could also stand some improvement. After a drug is released, the FDA monitors reports of problems with the drug and regulates the quality of its manufacture. Drug sales representatives are prohibited from promoting unapproved uses of drugs, although this protection did not work in the case of Natrecor. Drug representatives are also limited in what favors they can provide for doctors, to avoid inappropriate influence. Organizations like the American Medical Association issue ethical guidelines that companies usually follow voluntarily.

The system will always be imperfect, since regulations cannot address every problem. Pharmaceutical companies will always control what research they choose to do themselves. Controlling research questions limits the possible answers. Drug companies also decide, within the limits of regulation, what information to present to doctors and to the public. This control of information influences what medications doctors prescribe, unless doctors search out independent information and refuse to rely on pharmaceutical representatives and advertising.

Although regulations do not prevent inappropriate actions, they are at least an attempt to protect the public while allowing a degree of freedom and personal responsibility. By and large, the system is reasonably effective, so that the United States still provides most of the major medical

A Christian Perspective

In Matthew 23, Jesus criticizes the Pharisees for following little rules and missing big principles:

Woe to you, scribes and Pharisees, hypocrites! For you tithe mint and dill and cumin [people were required to give a percentage of their produce to the temple, and mint, dill, and cumin were tiny herbs], and have neglected the weightier provisions of the law: justice and mercy and faithfulness; but these are the things you should have done without neglecting the others. You blind guides, who strain out a gnat and swallow a camel! (Matt. 23:23–24)

Although they followed the letter of the regulations, they failed to follow its spirit. They made the minimum required donations to the temple and lived like the devil when it came to their fellow human beings. Their conduct was a lot like that of the twenty-first-century United States, except that the Pharisees paid more attention to the letter of the law than most of us do.

If Jesus had been a mortal legislator instead of a divine itinerant preacher, he might have approached the problem of the Pharisees the way our society does, by legislating behavior more precisely, requiring, for example, that a larger percentage of people's income go to the poor. Instead, Jesus appealed to a higher standard. He admonished them for not following the spirit of the law and appealed to them to fulfill the higher principles of justice and mercy and faith.

The goal for Christians is to exceed the requirements of the law and demonstrate the highest possible standards of selfless conduct. In a speech by Jesus called the Sermon on the Mount, he discusses the laws given to the people of Israel through Moses and in each case points to a higher standard. For example, he says:

> You have heard that the ancients were told, "You shall not commit murder" and "Whoever commits murder shall be liable to the court." But I say to you that everyone who is angry with his brother shall be guilty before the court; and whoever says to his brother, "You good-for-nothing," shall be guilty before the supreme court; and whoever says, "You fool," shall be guilty enough to go into the fiery hell. (Matt. 5:21–22)

In this sermon, Jesus draws a contrast between following the letter of the law and following the spirit of the law. Following the letter of the law is finding the narrowest possible interpretation and considering yourself acceptable if you fulfill that interpretation. In this example, it means not murdering someone. Following the spirit of the law means obeying the principle behind the law that goes beyond the limited prohibitions on a particular behavior. In this example, following the spirit of the law means having love for your brother and not having hatred, or even inappropriate anger. It goes even beyond actions to the level of attitudes and thoughts. This is an impossible standard apart from the grace of God. It requires dependence on his strength rather than human strength.

advances in the world and is still the major destination for foreign dignitaries seeking the best care.

High Ethical Standards versus Regulations: A Historical Perspective

Unfortunately, the weakening of our ethical values may destroy the supremacy of American medicine. It was over forty years ago now that President Kennedy received thunderous applause for his admonition "Ask not what your country can do for you, but ask what you can do for your country."[21] In contrast, now even the U.S. military uses recruiting slogans like "Be all you can be."[22] The focus now is on self, so that some have called this the "me generation."

In a society committed to truthfulness, self-sacrifice, and responsibility, people treat each other properly without any laws. In a society that focuses on following the letter of the law to individual advantage, extensive regulation is needed but will ultimately fail, since loopholes can always be found. The result is increased regulation, decreased personal freedom, and decreased cooperation.

In medicine, studies to assess the safety and efficacy of new treatments depend on doctors enrolling patients in trials. The doctor must choose to subject new treatments to such trials, rather than selling them without testing. The patient must also choose to participate in trials of new treatments, believing that the doctors are accurately disclosing the potential risks and benefits. The patient must choose to accept some risk, not only potentially to help himself but also to help others with the same condition. Without this trust and sacrifice, medicine cannot advance. Being overly trusting can subject us to harm. But loss of all trust and sacrifice will actually prevent medical progress.

Summary

In chapter 6, we learned that everyone is subject to bias. In this chapter, we have seen how bias affects doctors and drug companies. We have also seen how a number of protections against bias have been built into the system.

The first protection against bias is the scientific method. Using observation rather than reason allowed tremendous progress in medicine, so that we *know* what methods of diagnosis and treatment are effective. The same principles of science allow us to assess new treatments without being fooled by how smart we think we are. Scientific standards in the pharmaceutical industry help to ensure objective evaluation of new products.

The second protection against bias is the doctor. The selection and training of doctors encourages critical thinking, self-sacrifice, honesty, thoroughness, and knowledge. Some doctors abuse the trust they receive, but most try to fulfill their duty to their patients. Standards of treatment, objective data, clinical guidelines, ethical standards, and a desire for a good reputation all give the doctor a vested interest in treating her patients well, which usually offsets the temptations to compromise.

The third protection is regulation by government agencies and other organizations such as professional societies and insurance companies. In addition to actual regulation, fear of litigation provides an important motivator of objectivity. While imperfect, regulation has helped ensure that Americans have a health-care system that is among the best in the world.

The fourth protection is you, the consumer. You have a right and a responsibility to understand the rationale for treatments that are recommended. You are in a unique position to evaluate the character and competence of your physician. You bring your own values and perspective to your personal health-care concerns. Asking appropriate questions about tests and treatments allows you to discern the strengths and weaknesses of the approaches your doctor recommends. It also forces the doctor to think through the rationale for her recommendations and thereby helps protect you from your doctor's biases.

In the next section, you will see a part of the health-care continent where the first three protections are gone. In complementary and alternative medicine, science is often abandoned, the physician is left out, and government regulations have been rendered ineffective. We will look at this realm in detail, and I will give you the tools you need to protect yourself and your loved ones.

Notes

1. Thomas H. Lee and Troyen A. Brennan, "Direct-to-Consumer Marketing of High-Technology Screening Tests," *New England Journal of Medicine* 346 (2002): 529–31.

2. James H. Ehrlich, John A. Rumberger, and Alan G. Wasserman, letter to the editor, *New England Journal of Medicine* 346 (2002): 2010–13.

3. H. Gilbert Welch, *Should I Be Tested for Cancer? Maybe Not and Here's Why* (Berkeley: University of California Press, 2004).

4. Michael F. Roizen and Mehmet Oz, *You: The Smart Patient—An Insider's Handbook for Getting the Best Treatment* (New York: Free Press, 2006).

5. Claire Bombardier et al., "Comparison of Upper Gastrointestinal Toxicity of Rofecoxib and Naproxen in Patients with Rheumatoid Arthritis," *New England Journal of Medicine* 343 (2000): 1520–28.

6. Jeffrey M. Drazen, "Cox-2 Inhibitors: A Lesson in Unexpected Problems," *New England Journal of Medicine* 352 (2005): 1131–32.

7. Henry A. Waxman, "The Lessons of Vioxx: Drug Safety and Sales," *New England Journal of Medicine* 325 (2005): 2576–78.

8. Ibid.

9. Drazen, "Cox-2 Inhibitors."

10. Robert S. Bresalier et al., "Cardiovascular Events Associated with Rofecoxib in a Colorectal Adenoma Chemoprevention Trial," *New England Journal of Medicine* 352 (2005): 1092–102.

11. "Vioxx: An Unequal Partnership between Safety and Efficacy," unsigned editorial, *Lancet* 364 (2004): 1287–88.

12. Richard Horton, "Vioxx, the Implosion at Merck, and Aftershocks at the FDA," *Lancet* 364 (2004): 1995–96.

13. Joseph S. Alpert, "The Vioxx Debacle," *American Journal of Medicine* 118 (2005): 203–4.

14. Waxman, "Lessons of Vioxx."

15. Eric J. Topol, "Nesiritide—Not Verified," *New England Journal of Medicine* 352 (2005): 113–16.

16. Ibid.

17. Ibid.

18. "Ethics of Reciprocity," Wikipedia, http://en.wikipedia.org/wiki/Ethic_of_reciprocity (accessed June 17, 2006).

19. John F. Kennedy, "Radio and Television Report to the American People on Civil Rights," June 11, 1963, www.jfklibrary.org/Historical+Resources/Archives/Reference+Desk/Speeches/JFK/ 003POF03CivilRights06111963.htm (accessed June 17, 2006).

20. The Collected Works of Abraham Lincoln, ed. Roy P. Basler (August 1, 1858), 2:532, quoted in "A Collection of Abraham Lincoln Quotes," http://home.att.net/~rjnorton/Lincoln78.html (accessed June 17, 2006).

21. John F. Kennedy, inaugural address, 1961, www.bartleby.com/59/12/asknotwhatyo.html (accessed July 3, 2006).

22. Quoted in Frank M. Ahearn, "Be All You Can Be and Other Great American Slogans," 2004, www.peace.ca/beallyoucanbe.htm (accessed July 3, 2006).

PART 3

✚

ALTERNATIVE MEDICINE

8

✚

Is Alternative Medicine Better Than Conventional Medicine?

"Dr. Brown, we have talked a lot of about doctors and the scientific issues of medicine," said Julie. "But we still haven't discussed my supplements. As I said earlier, my friends tell me that medicines are dangerous but that if I'll just take these natural supplements I bought at the health food store, I will get well."

I turn back to her shopping bag with the twenty bottles in it. As I begin to remove them from the bag, I ask, "What makes you think that these things are safer than medications that are prescribed?"

"Well, Dr. Brown, these things are natural. Natural things can't hurt you, can they?"

What basis does Julie invoke for deciding the safety of these supplements? Is it reason, or is it the observation of truth in nature? Is reason a good way to determine truth? Is there any basis for believing that "natural is better"? Is there any basis for drawing a distinction between substances that are labeled "natural" and those that are labeled "pharmaceutical"?

The Problem with Reason

When I was an intern in St. Louis, I heard a story about another trainee in our program. As residents in training in internal medicine, we were responsible for the care of patients who suffered cardiac arrest. Therefore, when a "code" was called anywhere in the hospital, we would run to that location. A second- or third-year resident was in charge of the code and responsible for giving orders that the other members of the team obeyed. In general, the resident had never seen the patient before and had to quickly gather as much information as possible by talking to the nurses and any physicians present who had cared for the patient. This was a daunting responsibility for a doctor who had completed only one full year of training after medical school.

One day, a code was called on the orthopedics floor. The patient involved was a few days out from hip replacement surgery. She had complained of shortness of breath and had then collapsed. When my colleague arrived, the monitor showed that her heart was beating, but her blood pressure was undetectable.

Many patients who have hip surgery develop clots in their legs that can travel to the lungs. When this occurs, the patient will often become short of breath and may then have a cardiac arrest like this patient, with no blood pressure even though the heart is beating. My colleague concluded that the patient had suffered a blood clot to the lungs. This assumption made sense and needed to be seriously considered. Based on his belief that the patient had suffered a blood clot, he ordered that she be given a blood thinner. Unfortunately, as her autopsy later showed, her actual problem was not a blood clot at all. Instead, she had suffered massive internal bleeding, which was then aggravated by the blood thinner.

This story illustrates the problem with good ideas: they can be wrong. When our reasonable assumptions prove to be wrong, it is because not all of the facts were available or some of the available facts were not considered. Sometimes the thinker lacks the necessary perspective to reach the right conclusion. There may be something that the thinker does not even know to consider. Shakespeare articulates this problem through Hamlet: "There are more things in heaven and earth . . . than are dreamt of in your philosophy."[1]

In my earlier discussion of the history of science, we saw that the use of reason to determine truth took us nowhere. For thousands of years, medical care, science, and technology made no meaningful progress. When we opened our eyes and asked for the facts rather believing our own ideas, progress started. Since then, scientific knowledge has exploded, and our lives are better as a result. So let's open our eyes and look at the facts.

What Is "Natural"?

"Julie, how would you define *natural*?"

As I looked through her bag of supplements, it was hard to understand what anyone could feel was natural about them. They all looked like any other pills, except that a lot of them were larger than conventional medicine pills.

"Diet and exercise are certainly natural," Julie pointed out. "I guess that pills that contain things that are in our diet anyway would be natural. Things like vitamins and minerals."

"I would certainly agree that diet and exercise are natural. But if you take in a massive quantity of a substance that is in a food, a quantity you would never take in if you just ate the food, is it natural anymore? Garlic is a wonderful food that I greatly enjoy, but when I cook with garlic, I use it in fairly small quantities. If you take enough garlic to choke a horse and cram it into a pill, is that still natural? Vitamins are natural substances that have been shown to be necessary in small quantities for normal bodily function, but in excessive doses they can be harmful. Vitamin A, for example, can cause liver damage in high doses. Anyway, arsenic and hemlock are natural, too, and they kill people."

"I guess you're right."

I've just introduced Julie to several ideas that are new to her. Let's break these down into some basic concepts.

All Drugs Are Poisons

To carve a wooden sculpture, I need a knife sharp enough to cut the wood. Unfortunately, if the knife is sharp enough to cut the wood, it will also be sharp enough to cut my hand. Therefore, to carve a sculpture I must accept some risk of hurting myself. In the same way, any treatment strong enough to change the way my body functions in a *positive* way will also have some potential to affect my body in a *negative* way. To receive a *benefit* from a treatment, I accept some risk of a *negative effect* from that treatment.

On my bookshelf sits a huge book called *The Physician's Desk Reference* (PDR). It contains an entry for every prescription drug available. For each drug, there are a number of sections that explain how the drug works, what conditions it treats, and what potential adverse effects are associated with it. So far, I have never looked up a drug and seen the entry under potential adverse effects to be "none." Every drug has potential adverse effects. The real questions are, What *are* the potential adverse effects? How often do they happen? Are they reversible?

The risks and side effects of drugs vary depending on the condition being treated and the availability of alternatives. On one extreme, medicines for high blood pressure have side effects only rarely, or the drug never makes it to market. On the other extreme, chemotherapy, while better than it once was, is often associated with severe side effects. Most drugs are somewhere in between. Doctors and patients weigh the potential side effects against the potential benefits and decide what treatment makes the most sense. Unfortunately, sometimes a drug has more adverse effects than we know when it is first released.

In chapter 6, we discussed the process by which a drug gets to the market. You may remember that after the drug is on the market, there is "after-marketing surveillance," a system by which the FDA is informed of adverse events that happen to people taking a medication. The doctor reporting the events is not supposed to decide whether or not the drug is responsible; instead doctors are to report everything bad that happens to someone who has begun to take the medication. Then, if the same event is reported in Texas and Nebraska and Oregon, someone will recognize that there is a problem. Through this process, drugs are often removed from the market six months after their release, generally because of the discovery of a rare but serious side effect. For example, if a drug to treat high blood pressure kills one person out of 10,000, that risk is unacceptable, since hypertension is not an immediately life-threatening problem and there are many drugs to treat it with a lower risk of fatality.

As a rule, more potent drugs are more toxic. For example, we have strong medications that break up blood clots in people having heart attacks. Since they *break up* blood clots, they can cause severe bleeding in someone who has recently had surgery. We have milder drugs that *prevent the formation* of new clots but do not break up existing clots. The risk of bleeding with these drugs is lower: they will have little effect on surgical sites that have had time to heal. However, they are less effective in the case of a heart attack, since they do not break up an existing clot. To expect a drug to be stronger but also less toxic would be nonsensical. If a knife is sharper, it will be easier to cut yourself.

Julie's friends have told her that the pills from the health food store will "make her well" whereas my pills can only help her heart get stronger. Somehow, however, they claim that these very potent supplements have no risk of toxicity. To hear her friends talk, you would expect that if these products had an entry in the PDR, the "potential adverse effects" section would read simply "none."

Why don't these products have an entry in the PDR? That brings us to the next principle.

Natural Products Are Drugs

Prior to the twentieth century, most drugs were made from plants. We now refer to these drugs as "botanicals." Most botanicals have been abandoned as worthless or harmful. One exception in cardiology is a drug called digitalis, made from the purple foxglove. The leaves of the plant contain the active ingredient. Digitalis is used to control heart rate in a condition called atrial fibrillation and also has modest beneficial effects in congestive heart failure.

Does every ingredient in the leaf of the plant help patients with these conditions? Is the amount of the ingredient the same in every purple foxglove leaf, in every plant, in every season? The answer to both questions is a resounding no. These questions get at the central problem with botanicals: safety and efficacy. This issue is particularly critical with digitalis. If someone receives just a little more digitalis than the effective dose, the drug can kill them. People today still die of digitalis toxicity, usually because of accidental over-dose. If I learn how many leaves to use to treat a patient one year, and the next year the plant receives more rain or less sunlight, how will the number of leaves needed change? Should I use more leaves or fewer leaves? I guess if some-one dies, I'll know I used too many leaves. Of course, if I use too few leaves, the medicine will not help the person. Do you want me to have to figure out the right dose each season by testing it in patients like you?

Today, scientists can separate the ingredients in foxglove leaves and demonstrate which components are helpful and which are harmful. The active ingredient can be purified and dosed properly, year in and year out. Is it safer to take the whole leaf because somehow this seems more natural, or is it safer to take the purified active ingredient?

The issue of safety and efficacy is the same, whether the product is labeled "natural" or not. If anything, when a combination of substances is used together, the chances of toxicity are worse: whole plants are even more prob-lematic than isolated ingredients.

Today, some supplements are made from whole plants and have the problems outlined above. Others, however, are individual chemicals isolated from plants. In that case, how can anyone argue that they are different from substances that are called "drugs"? Intellectually and logically, there is no basis for drawing a distinction. Unfortunately, there is a *legal* distinction.

A Market Explosion

When I was a child, use of herbal remedies was a fringe practice in U.S. society. Health food stores were rare. They seemed to be part of a countercultural movement against "the establishment." Today, mainline drugstores contain sections with natural remedies, and health food stores are owned by people who wear business suits and drive fancy cars. What changed? Was it some great revelation that many unconventional medications could cure disease where conventional medications had failed?

Unfortunately, the change did not occur because of some great scientific revelation. Instead, it occurred because of a change in the law. In 1994, President Bill Clinton signed the Dietary Supplement Health and Education Act (DSHEA). This act defined *supplement* as a product "intended to supplement the diet that bears or contains one or more of the following dietary ingredients: a vitamin, a mineral, an herb or other botanical, an amino acid, a dietary substance . . . or a concentrate, metabolite, extract, or combinations of these ingredients."[2] The act exempted supplements from the premarket safety evaluations required of food ingredients. Therefore, these products now are less regulated than food and food additives. While the act forbids claims that a supplement can treat a disease, this requirement is easily circumvented. For example, a supplement cannot bear a label stating that it "treats arthritis," but it can say that it "promotes joint health."

Supplement manufacturers do not have to prove that their products are safe or effective. This led to an explosion in the industry, so that as of 2001, almost $18 billion was spent on supplements in the United States.[3] Traditional drug-store chains couldn't resist getting a piece of the pie, and supplements are now sold everywhere.

Since the purveyors of these products do not have to prove safety or efficacy, what protection remains? The FDA can act only if there is a "significant or unreasonable risk of illness of injury."[4] With medications that go through the approval process for a drug, the presumption is that the substance is neither safe nor effective, and the manufacturer has to prove that it is useful and not harmful.

For the government, food additives are a separate category. Food dyes, for example, are additives. Additives are assumed to be harmful, and the manufacturer has to prove that the product is safe. If questions of safety arise later, it is fairly easy for the FDA to take the product off the market, as it has in recent years with certain dyes.

"Supplements," in contrast to "drugs" or "additives," are assumed to be safe, and the *government* would have to prove that they are *unsafe*. As we will see in the next chapter, getting these products off the market is very difficult. In 2002, for example, the FDA issued warnings about potential liver toxicity, kidney toxicity, and cancer-causing potential of products containing kava, comfrey, and arostolochic acid, but all of these products are still on the market.[5]

In chapters 6 and 7 we discussed the problem of bias and the fact that all of us have biases. It is important to recognize these and protect ourselves from them. I reviewed the slow, multistep process by which a drug gains FDA approval and showed how safeguards are built in to prevent bias. In addition to governmental regulation, doctors expect to see publication of research results in reputable journals before they prescribe a medication. Despite these protections, harm sometimes occurs.

Contrast this system to the market for supplements. There are no meaningful limits on what a manufacturer can claim about the products. With an article suggesting why the product might be helpful, a few testimonials, and some nice packaging, they're in business. You are at the mercy of the ethics of the manufacturer. Unless you seek it out, you have no input from a doctor. And unlike conventional medicine, there is no mandatory after-market surveillance for adverse events.

If you had to fly somewhere, would you rather climb aboard a jet operated by one of the airlines or climb into the helicopter my Uncle Albert built in his garage? The contrast in the risk involved and the trust required is just as great when you consider regulated drugs versus unregulated supplements.

Supplements Should Be Held to the Same Standard as Other Drugs

Since all drugs are poisons and natural products are drugs, natural products are also poisons and should be held to the same standard as other drugs. Unfortunately, that industry and its adherents often assert that proof of safety and efficacy is not necessary. In an excellent article in the *New England Journal of Medicine* in 1998, Marcia Angell and Jerome Kassirer point out that "what most sets alternative medicine apart, in our view, is that it has not been scientifically tested and its advocates largely deny the need for such testing."[6] They conclude:

> It is time for the scientific community to stop giving alternative medicine a free ride. There cannot be two kinds of medicine —conventional and alternative. There is only medicine that has been adequately tested and medicine that

A Christian Perspective

Does Christianity have anything to say about these competitive views of medicine? Is one approach more consistent with a Christian worldview?

As we discussed in chapter 5, Christianity and modern science both evaluate truth by examining an external standard. Rather than relying on biased reason, science answers medical questions by careful observation in nature. Rather than relying on biased reason, Christianity answers moral questions by examining the Bible. As documented in chapter 5, many of the leaders of the scientific revolution stated explicitly that their approach to science was rooted in the biblical belief that God reveals truth in the world of nature, and that human reason is inferior to this revelation.

In contrast, advertisements promoting alternative medicine often rely on reason and subjective experience. Some alternative practitioners argue that ancient views of health and disease from other cultures are just as valid as our own, and do not need to meet our standards of scientific proof. (As noted above, in the physical sciences, the value of an idea is unequivocally obvious when subjected to experimentation, so that this argument carries no weight.) The rejection of an external standard is analogous to New Age spirituality, which accepts a multitude of different belief systems as equally valid. Of course, this viewpoint is not universal in alternative medicine. Some alternative practitioners do try to assess their treatments scientifically. However, those who do not accept the importance of scientific evaluation are on the slippery slope of subjectivity.

has not, medicine that works and medicine that may or may not work. Once a treatment has been tested rigorously, it no longer matters whether it was considered alternative at the outset. If it is found to be reasonably safe and effective, it will be accepted. But assertions, speculation, and testimonials do not substitute for evidence. Alternative treatments should be subjected to scientific testing no less rigorous than that required for conventional treatments.[7]

If I am going to take a substance into my body, I want to have reasonable assurance that it may help my illness. I also want to know what risks are associated with its use. You should have that same standard for your family.

So far I have focused on supplements and contrasted their lack of regulation to the FDA's strict regulation of drugs. Conventional medical treatments that do not involve drugs are also studied scientifically before their general adoption by the medical community. These treatments would include physical therapy, medical devices, and operations. In contrast, a number of alternative, nonmedication therapies have not been subjected to such testing, but they should be before they are accepted as safe or effective. Such alternative therapies include magnets, therapeutic touch, copper bracelets, and a host of others.

A Worldview Perspective

Prior to the 1960s, the predominant worldview in the United States assumed the existence of good and evil, right and wrong, truth and falsehood. Now, in what has been called the postmodern worldview, many people believe that there is no right and wrong. There are things that are true for me and not true for you. If you want to believe something different from what I believe, who am I to tell you that you're wrong? This worldview, this belief system, has come to dominate American thought about morality and religion.

For obvious reasons, this worldview has made little progress in the world of the physical sciences. If you build an airplane based on rules of physics you have made up for yourself, it will not get off the ground. However, postmodernism has affected the way we deal with new concepts in all other areas of academics. Most of mainstream society today is hesitant to tell anyone that their ideas are wrong.

It is this attitude of accommodation that has led to the very term *complementary and alternative medicine*. There is no evidence that it *complements* traditional medicine. Indeed, the potential for adverse interactions between supplements and prescription drugs is serious. There is also no scientific evidence that these treatments as a group provide a viable *alternative* to conventional medicine. While some individual treatments may be effective, we do not conclude that they are effective because they belong to this group. To be proved effective, they must be tested in the same way as conventional medicines. The term *complementary and alternative medicine* is politically correct: it pretends that conventional medicine and unconventional medicine are the same, that both are equally true, and that both exist together in one big, happy family.

Are the biological sciences somehow different from the physical sciences? The experiences of the past hundred years shout that they are not. The use of reason without data has repeatedly led to failure in medicine, and the use of careful observation has led to a revolution that has prolonged the average lifespan by thirty years since the beginning of the twentieth century. If we abandon the scientific method and replace it with reason and tradition without adequate testing, we are returning to the Dark Ages.

Summary

"So, Julie, your choice is not between 'harmless, life-saving natural herbs' and 'dangerous drugs.' Your choice is between two sets of drugs. One set of drugs has been carefully studied in thousands of people like you. There are risks associated with them, but we know what those risks are. For you, the risks of taking medications are far less than the risks of not taking them. The other choice is a set of drugs that, as a group, has not been adequately studied but is being sold without proof of safety or efficacy. I know that you can find well-written articles about the good ideas behind these products. There are good ideas behind the prescription medications, too. But more important, prescription drugs do not rely on ideas alone. They have been tested and shown to help."

Notes

1. William Shakespeare, *Hamlet, Prince of Denmark*, c. 1601, act 1, scene 5.

2. Food and Drug Administration, "Dietary Supplement Health and Education Act of 1994," December 1, 1995, http://vm.cfsan.fda.gov/~dms/dietsupp.html (accessed September 7, 2005).

3. Donald M. Marcus and Arthur P. Grollman, "Botanical Medicines: The Need for New Regulations," *New England Journal of Medicine* 347 (2002): 2073–76.

4. Food and Drug Administration, "Dietary Supplement."

5. Marcus and Grollman, "Botanical Medicine."

6. Marcia Angell and Jerome P. Kassirer, "Alternative Medicine: The Risks of Untested and Unregulated Remedies," *New England Journal of Medicine* 339 (1998): 839–41.

7. Ibid., 841.

9

✚

Dying of Natural Causes

Alternative Medicines Aren't Dangerous, Are They?

"Dr. Brown," Julie responded, "I understand what you are saying. It makes sense that any substance we take into our body that can help us will also have the potential to cause harm, whether it is called natural or not. But natural supplements haven't hurt anyone, have they?"

"Julie, I wish that were true. There are a number of examples we will discuss."

"But the people who sell these products claim that studies prove they help people like me. Are these people lying?"

"What a study actually means depends on a lot of factors. Usually, one study alone does not establish the truth about a treatment. It is important that the studies ask the right questions. They also need to be done with proper methods and large numbers of patients. Let me give you some examples to show you what I mean."

The Disappointing Story of Antioxidants

After breakfast, Cindy opened each of the three bottles beside her sink and extracted a pill. She then downed the vitamin E, vitamin C, and beta-carotene. She had watched her mother die of colon cancer, and she was going to be sure that she avoided that fate. She knew that antioxidants would protect her.

For decades, scientists have known that the body handles bad molecules, such as waste products and contaminants, by using *oxidation*, which involves giving these bad molecules an extra electron. The extra electron sticks out like a knife. These dangerously armed bad molecules, now known as *free radicals*, are dismantled quickly by other molecules called *antioxidants*. The antioxidants grab the protruding knives and stab them into garbage receptacles. If the antioxidants don't get to them fast enough, the knives can damage normal tissues. In reality, the antioxidants get rid of the free radicals quite rapidly, so that at any given time there are not many free radicals around, and most of the damage they do is quickly repaired. However, scientists have long suspected that small amounts of unrepaired damage might accumulate and lead to disease and deterioration.

Fifty years ago, researchers suggested that taking extra antioxidants in the diet would help disarm these bandits faster and therefore reduce the risk of cancer, heart attack, and stroke. It might even slow down the aging process, so the theory went.

A number of studies looked at the relationship between intake of foods containing antioxidants and the risk of cancer. They found that those who took in large amounts of antioxidants *in their food* had less cancer risk. This is called an *observational study*, because the researchers just observe what happens without interfering.

Is that the right experiment? If you want to know if taking antioxidants as *pills* will help, it is only a good place to start. It is not the right final experiment. Fruits and vegetables are the primary dietary source of antioxidants. Therefore, people who take in a lot of antioxidants are eating a healthy diet. People who eat a healthy diet may be at reduced risk for having cancer, but not necessarily because of the antioxidants.

If you really want to know if antioxidant pills reduce cancer risk, you start with two groups of people who follow similar diets. You give one group antioxidant pills. The other group gets a pill that looks the same but contains no antioxidants. Then, watch to see what happens. If the group taking the antioxidants does better, the antioxidants are helpful. If the group getting antioxidants does not do better, the antioxidants are not helping. Multiple trials like this have now been completed.

In October 2004, a review was published examining the data from fourteen randomized trials that asked whether antioxidants would reduce the risk of getting cancers of the digestive tract. In total, 170,525 people were enrolled in these studies.[1]

Not only did these studies show no reduction in cancer risk, they showed an increase in the risk of death in those taking antioxidants. Did you catch that? Not only did the supplements fail to help, they could kill you. The authors calculated that 0.9 percent, or almost 1 percent, of people who use antioxidant supplements will *die earlier than they would have without the supplements*.[2] What this means is that if you take antioxidants, the best you can hope for is that you have wasted your money. There is no evidence that the pills will help with anything. In addition to having no benefit, there is a 1 percent chance that you will die early. If there were a prescription drug with no benefits and a 1 percent risk of early death, it would be taken off the market immediately.

Why were scientists wrong about antioxidants? It was a great idea. That is not enough. There were large studies asking *preliminary* questions that suggested benefit. That is not enough either. Small randomized trials asking the right question also showed benefit. But small studies are not enough either. When large studies were done, there was no benefit. And when a review looked at multiple studies in aggregate, there was evidence of harm. Now, to be fair, this report is not definitive either, since it combined different treatments, but its results are very worrisome.

Has the supplement industry stopped claiming that antioxidants prevent cancer? Fire up your computer and look on the Internet to find out. I think you already know the answer. You cannot rely on purveyors of these products to provide adverse information from the medical literature. Like all of us, they are human and biased.

The story with the antioxidant vitamin E and heart disease is similar. Observational studies suggested that vitamin E helped, but when randomized trials were done, they showed that vitamin E does not help. Many cardiologists recommended the use of vitamin E in the 1990s based on observational studies. Hopefully, those who did recognized that they were doing so based on preliminary data and informed their patients that the benefits were uncertain. A study published in 2005 showed no reduction in the risk of heart attack, stroke, or cancer but showed an increase in the risk of congestive heart failure.[3] Therefore, once again, a good idea that appeared to work turned out to be harmful instead.

The experience with vitamin E also demonstrates the difficulties in interpreting the results of research. Even physicians, who are trained to be skeptical, decided to proceed with therapies that later turned out to be harmful. You should not rely on your own opinion or the opinions of those who sell supplements. The best you can do is to rely on your doctor or other independent sources of information. Your doctor may still turn out to be wrong, but she is better trained to accurately evaluate the available information accurately.

Your doctor does represent a reasonably independent source of information. Contrary to the allegations of some in the alternative industry, doctors do not make less money if they offer a positive opinion about supplements. Indeed, given the popularity of supplements, doctors stand to gain by endorsing these products. Frequently, ads for alternative products appear in physician magazines. The heading on the ads is not "Save lives! Prevent disease!" Instead, the heading on the ads is "Increase your income!" If anything, doctors stand to lose popularity by taking a strong stand against alternative products. Having said this, your doctor is the one person whose sole responsibility is to you as the patient and who does not have a vested interest in what approach you choose.

In summary, antioxidants have failed. Even though they are natural, even though they seemed like a good idea, and even though initial studies suggested that they help, they turned out to be harmful, although the risks were small statistically and therefore hard to see. In the next case, you will see severe and very visible harm from a supplement.

L-Tryptophan and the Eosinophilia-Myalgia Syndrome

Christine loved her job. Even though international travel had lost some of its thrill, she loved selling her company's products in Europe, Asia, and even Africa. The one thing she never got used to was jet lag. She was ecstatic to learn about L-tryptophan, an amino acid some scientists believed was part of the normal signal used by the body to get the brain to sleep. She started using it faithfully when she crossed time zones, and it seemed to help. She needed to recover from her trip quickly when she arrived on the other side of the world.

One day, she noticed that she was having a hard time getting up off the toilet. Instead of just standing up easily, she had to use her arms to pull herself up. As she began her journey back to the States a few days later, she noticed that it was hard to carry her luggage, even hard to walk without stopping to rest every ten yards. When she arrived in Albuquerque, she was beginning to feel out of breath. Her family took her straight to the hospital.

L-tryptophan is an amino acid. It is a part of every protein in our bodies. Beginning in the 1970s, it was marketed in supplement form as a treatment not only for insomnia but also for premenstrual tension, stress, pain, weight loss, and depression.[4]

Late on Tuesday afternoon, November 7, 1989, a field investigator for the FDA in New Mexico telephoned FDA headquarters with disturbing news. A new medical condition had appeared. People were developing fever, fatigue, shortness of breath, cough, joint pains, and severe muscle aches. Some of them had developed nerve problems that led to paralysis and even failure of their ability to breathe, so that they had to be placed on breathing machines. The disease also caused memory loss and difficulty in thinking.[5]

Thirty cases had been reported, but no one had died at that point. The investigator suspected that L-tryptophan might be responsible.[6]

On November 11, a warning was issued to the public, and on November 17, the FDA requested a nationwide recall of all over-the-counter dietary supplements containing 100 mg or more of L-tryptophan. On March 23, 1990, all marketed products containing any L-tryptophan at all were recalled.[7]

By 1991, doctors had reported 1,500 cases and 31 deaths. It is now believed that the final number was far larger. In those individuals who survived, most got better, with the exception of those who had nerve damage; they either stayed the same or got worse.[8] Many people were either killed or permanently disabled by this drug.

There is an interesting epilogue to this story. Manufacturers produced L-tryptophan by growing bacteria in vats, then extracting the product from the bacteria. In order to make the process cheaper, the leading supplier created genetically altered bacteria to produce much larger amounts of L-tryptophan. Consequently, a new contaminant was present in tiny amounts in the finished product. This contaminant was actually two molecules of L-tryptophan that were chemically stuck together into a single molecule. As it turned out, this contaminant was responsible for all of the death and destruction.[9]

There are some frightening possibilities if we consider what could have happened. What if the contaminant had been present in the pills from a small company instead of a large one, so that there were fewer cases and the problem escaped detection? How do we know that this has not happened with other products? What if the people who came in with paralysis had denied taking any medicines, since they thought L-tryptophan was not a medicine?

The scariest question, however, is, what if this had happened after 1994, when the law changed, making it harder and slower to get dangerous supplements off the market? The story of ephedra answers that question.

Ephedra

Bill had decided it was time lose weight. At thirty-nine and with three small children, he wanted to be around to care for his family. He loved his wife, and nothing gave him more joy than holding his children on his lap and reading to them at night.

His friend Greg had recently lost twenty pounds.

"How did you do it, Greg?"

"Mostly it was diet and exercise. I tried to eat about half what I was used to eating, and I started walking and jogging for about half an hour each evening."

"Didn't you starve?"

"Well, I probably would have, but a friend gave me these natural pills that helped me lose weight. They seemed to curb my appetite, although sometimes they seemed to make my heart race."

"Are they dangerous?"

"How could they be? They're natural. It's not like they're drugs. Here, I have some left. Why don't you try them?"

Bill accepted the pills and immediately swallowed two of them. After work that day, Bill put on his sweat suit and tennis shoes. He kissed his wife and children goodbye and told them he would be back in half an hour. After walking a block, he felt his heart racing. He also noticed he was out of breath.

"Maybe that's what Greg was talking about when he said these pills made his heart race."

As he continued to walk, the heart racing seemed faster, and it got even harder to breathe. He began to feel light-headed, as if he might pass out. Gradually, he realized that he was in trouble and needed help.

"If I can just make it to the door at that next house," he thought.

As he started up the driveway, he finally couldn't walk anymore. Somehow, he managed to fall onto the grass instead of the concrete. As he lay there, the feelings got no better. Instead, he began to feel a great weight on his chest, as it got harder and harder to breathe. As he closed his eyes for the last time, he hoped that his wife and children would know that he had taken the pills and exercised today only because he loved them so much.

Adrenaline is the "fight or flight hormone." It is the substance that is released in your body when someone cuts you off in traffic, or when your alarm clock goes off, or when the doctor gives you bad news. You know that your adrenaline level has gone up because your heart beats harder and faster. You also may notice that you lose your appetite. As we will see, it is this latter property of adrenaline that has been exploited commercially, to help people lose weight.

When your adrenaline level goes up for a brief time, you fight harder and run faster ("the fight or flight" response). Unfortunately, adrenaline has harmful effects in the longer term if the level stays elevated. High adrenaline levels promote clot formation, which is a major factor in heart attacks. Adrenaline raises heart rate and blood pressure and stimulates abnormal heart rhythms that can lead to cardiac arrest and death.

As it turns out, there are a number of different compounds that act like adrenaline when taken into the body. Caffeine is a mild example. Many of these compounds, like caffeine, occur in nature. Others have been made synthetically. Since they have modest effects on decreasing appetite, such compounds have been tried to help people lose weight.

Drugs like this, whether prescription or "alternative," do decrease appetite *in the short term*. However, when you stop taking the drug, the effect is gone, and you regain the weight. In addition, in many cases, even if the drug is continued, the effects on appetite go away as the body becomes accustomed to the medication.

Unfortunately, ineffectiveness in the long term is not the only problem with these drugs. As you would expect from my description of adrenaline, these drugs are also highly toxic. In the case of prescription drugs, doctors are warned not to prescribe these products to people with heart trouble or high blood pressure, because the medications will raise heart rate and blood pressure.

Despite these warnings, some prescription drugs have been taken off the market in the United States due to toxicity. In 1997, the FDA took two adrenaline-like prescription drugs, fenfluramine and dexfenfluramine, off the market because they appeared to damage heart valves.[10] Doctors had already abandoned Dexfenfluramine because of reports that it might cause a serious and usually fatal disorder called pulmonary hypertension.[11] Again, these were prescription drugs, prescribed by doctors who were supposed to avoid their use in patients with heart disease or high blood pressure. Even in this context, two of these drugs proved so dangerous that they were taken off the market.

Into this notorious group of drugs came ephedra. Used in traditional Chinese medicine as a treatment for asthma (adrenaline-like substances are used for this purpose in traditional Western medicine as well), ephedra had been promoted for weight loss. It became increasingly recognized by doctors as a cause of abnormal heart rhythms, heart attack, and death. In March 2003, a report was published in the *Journal of the American Medical Association* reviewing the published literature to date on this drug and the closely related drug ephedrine.[12]

Was the drug helpful if used long term? No trials looked at the use of ephedra for more than six months. Did it even help for weight loss in the short term? In the short-term trials, the average patient lost a little more than a pound per month more with ephedra than with placebo. That is not much difference for people who are trying to lose a significant amount of weight. What adverse effects did the drug have? Not only did the drug have no meaningful effect on weight loss, but people who used the drug were 2.2–3.6 times as likely to have psychiatric problems, stomach problems, and heart palpitations.[13]

These investigators reviewed case reports of adverse events as well, including 71 published case reports, 1,820 case reports made to the FDA, and 15,951 reports of adverse events made to a single manufacturer of this drug. These reports noted five deaths, five heart attacks, eleven strokes, four seizures, and eight episodes of psychiatric problems related to these drugs.[14] Of course, *reported* deaths are often the tip of the iceberg: most people do not think that the death of their loved one could be due to something "natural" and so do not tell the doctor that their loved one was taking a supplement. As knowledge about ephedra spread, more deaths were reported. By 2004, 155 deaths had been reported.[15]

In the first part of this chapter, I discussed the case of L-tryptophan, where the FDA suspected a problem on Tuesday, issued a warning on Saturday, and initiated a recall the next Friday. That was before the law changed with the DSHEA in 1994. Now it is much harder to remove an alternative product from the market, since these products are heavily protected. Doctors had known for a long time before the paper in March 2003 that there was a problem.

With almost 16,000 adverse event reports, you should suspect that the manufacturers knew there was a problem, too. However, under the law, the FDA had to overcome tremendous hurdles to remove ephedra from the market.

Finally, on December 30, 2003, nine months after the publication in the *Journal of the American Medical Association*, the FDA issued a warning and requested that manufacturers stop making products containing ephedra. On February 11, 2004, the FDA issued a rule prohibiting the sale of these products. Two manufacturers went to court to block enforcement of the rule, so that the ban actually did not go into effect until April 12, 2004, more than a year after the journal article.[16]

Alternative Medicine Fights Back with New Alternative Medicines

As more information about the dangers of ephedra became available, the industry should have taken a cautious approach to its sale and been reluctant to produce a similar drug. But the supplement industry had no intention of giving up the huge market for weight-loss products. As the ban was being contemplated, industry leaders were already searching for the next ephedra. In April 2004, just after the ban on ephedra, an article appeared in *Forbes* magazine titled "Poison Pills: The Men and Money Pushing Dangerous Diet Supplements." In that article, Nathan Vardi tells the story of Robert Chinery Jr. Chinery had a company called Cytodyne Technologies. His company manufactured the ephedra-containing supplement found in the locker of Baltimore Oriole pitcher Steven Bechler, who died during spring training in 2003 with ephedra in his system. By October 2003, Vardi reports, Chinery had pushed his company into bankruptcy by selling off its assets to other entities that he partially owned. Since the company went bankrupt, it was no longer vulnerable to lawsuits.

At the time of the article, Chinery was marketing a weight-loss product that he described to customers as "ephedra free." This product contains "bitter orange," another adrenaline-like substance. Bitter orange is now used throughout the supplement industry and has become the next ephedra. If ephedra is an adrenaline-like substance and it kills people, will bitter orange be safe, though it is also like adrenaline? Chinery and his colleagues in this industry obviously do not care whether it is safe or not, since they are selling the product without appropriate scientific study.[17]

It's not just ephedra. *Consumer Reports* has had many articles through the years that paint supplements in a favorable light. In May 2004, however, it reported on twelve supplements that are known to carry risks such as cancer, liver failure, kidney failure, and death. Despite the fact that the FDA had issued warnings to the public about these products, the investigators were able to purchase them easily at stores and on the Internet.[18]

Do you still think that you can trust this industry? Then keep reading.

Deception

A few years ago, a supplement called PC-SPES appeared to show promise in the treatment of prostate cancer. Doctors were impressed with some preliminary data and decided to study this supplement more carefully. When the product was analyzed, it was found to contain, among other things, diethylstilbestrol, a form of estrogen, which is a female hormone.[19] Since one of the drug approaches to the treatment of prostate cancer is the suppression of testosterone, it makes sense that giving a female hormone

A Christian Perspective

As discussed in chapter 2, which looked at dishonesty among conventional doctors, each of us has the potential for evil. That potential is also present in purveyors of alternative treatments. We should not be surprised when some of them are dishonest.

Another principle in scripture is that we cannot expect to get something for nothing. When we try to get something for nothing, we are looking for trouble. The Bible warns us that "a faithful man will abound with blessings, but he who hastes to be rich will not go unpunished" (Prov. 28:20). This verse promises the benefits of faithful work but warns that those who try to take shortcuts to wealth will face consequences. Two verses later, we are told, "A man with an evil eye hastens after wealth and does not know that want will come upon him" (Prov. 28:22). That is, schemes to get rich quickly usually end in poverty rather than wealth.

While these proverbs refer to finances, the principle holds in other areas of life as well. If you want to lose weight, pills may help in the short run,

might be of some benefit. However, that was not what prostate cancer sufferers had in mind when they bought this "natural" substance that the manufacturers falsely claimed did not contain "drugs." Estrogen would obviously cause the development of sexual problems and female physical characteristics, such as the growth of breast tissue. It would also carry the risks that estrogens always carry, such as the development of life-threatening blood clots.

Contamination of supplements with drugs and poisons is not rare. The California Department of Health reported in 1998 that one-third of Asian patent medicines sold in that but in the long run, the weight will come back. If you want to lose weight and keep it off, changes in your diet and your exercise will be required. Do not expect a quick and easy solution; it is just not realistic. Similarly, if a cancer is growing in your body, it will not just go away because you eat a different diet. The idea that there is such an easy way out is naive.

We have an obligation to God to care for our bodies. Paul explains that our bodies are temples of the Holy Spirit and thus we are not our own (1 Cor. 6:19–20). Therefore, we should be careful about what we put into our bodies. We should not accept something as important as health advice from just anyone who happens to have a website.

Finally, from a Christian perspective, truth is determined by God's revelation in nature using the scientific method. There is not a separate standard of truth for things called "natural" and things called "pharmaceutical." Reason is inferior to observation as a method of determining what is effective in treating health problems.

state contained undeclared pharmaceuticals or poisonous heavy metals. The drugs contained in supplements in other studies included hormones, Viagra, tranquilizers, diabetes medicines, and fenfluramine.[20] A study of herbal medicines in Boston found dangerous levels of lead, mercury, and arsenic in 20 percent of the preparations tested.[21]

In chapter 7 we saw how conventional pharmaceutical companies sometimes make bad choices due to bias or due to greed. In this chapter we have seen that the supplement industry is often guilty of making bad choices. While some supplement companies try to be honest and responsible, others engage in deliberate deception.

A Worldview Perspective

The idea that alternative medicine products do not need regulation is based on the concept that they have no risk of harm. That idea is obviously wrong. Defining them legally as "foods" was a foolish mistake. Until this mistake is corrected, unscrupulous entrepreneurs will continue to exploit this loophole in order to make a fast buck. The industry has shamelessly deceived the public on multiple occasions and deserves to be strictly regulated for what it is: a "wild west" corner of the pharmaceutical industry.

For a consumer, it is naive to believe that there is some magical treatment that can cure a serious health problem without risk. It is still more naive to believe the lie that your doctor is ignorant of these miracle cures. While it is wise to explore options, it is foolish to do so without input from your personal physician.

Both conventional and alternative practitioners have the potential to be dishonest. In conventional medicine, there are a number of checks and balances in place that attempt to protect the consumer from deliberate abuse and from the bias in decision making that is always present when there is a conflict of interest. Unfortunately, such checks and balances were removed from the supplement industry by the changes in law that occurred with the DSHEA. In addition, those who give advice about supplements include salespeople and unregulated practitioners who do not have the strong tradition of self-sacrifice and honesty that is inculcated into conventional physicians (see chapter 3).

If an alternative medicine turns out to be effective based on strong evidence, conventional practitioners accept the proof of its treatments. Publication of both favorable and unfavorable trial results for alternative treatments in conventional medical journals demonstrates this commitment to truth. The early, widespread use of alternative treatments such as vitamin E, saw palmetto, and gingko by physicians also demonstrates openness to these approaches, even though later trials were disappointing.

Conventional practitioners will always have jobs, no matter what treatments turn out to work. However, purveyors of so-called natural remedies risk losing their livelihood if they tell you that their treatments are dangerous or ineffective, since they cannot offer conventional treatments. Without checks and balances to protect the consumer, there is no hope for consistent high-quality information within the supplement industry.

Protecting Yourself

As a physician, with rare exceptions, I do not prescribe even drugs that have passed the FDA approval process until they have been on the market for a year. In this way, I let other people find out the problems with new products. Supplements do not go through any approval process, and they have no mandatory reporting of adverse events. To justify the use of such substances to me, you need a very compelling reason and a lot of strong evidence.

In this chapter, we have looked at the issue of the *safety* of supplements and found that without proper testing, they cannot meet the standard of safety. In the next chapter, we will look at the issue of *effectiveness* and learn how to look critically at scientific evidence.

Notes

1. Goran Bjelakovic, Dimitrinka Nikolova, Rosa G. Simonetti, and Christian Gluud, "Antioxidant Supplements for Prevention of Gastrointestinal Cancers: A Systematic Review and Meta-analysis," *Lancet* 364 (2004): 1219–28.

2. Ibid.

3. HOPE and HOPE-TOO Trial Investigators, "Effects of Long-Term Vitamin E Supplementation on Cardiovascular Events and Cancer," *Journal of the American Medical Association* 293 (2005): 1338–47.

4. Douglas L. Archer, "Statement by Douglas L. Archer, Ph.D., Deputy Director, Center for Food Safety and Applied Nutrition, Food and Drug Administration, in Testimony before the Subcommittee on Human Resources and Intergovernmental Relations Committee, 18 July 1991," http://vm.cfscan.fda.gov/~dmsds-tryp2.html (accessed June 3, 2005).

5. Eugene Braunwald et al., eds., *Harrison's Principles of Internal Medicine*, 15th ed. (New York: McGraw-Hill, 2001), 1946.

6. Archer, "Statement."

7. Ibid.

8. Braunwald et al., *Harrison's Principles of Internal Medicine*.

9. John Fagan, "Summary of the Tryptophan Toxicity Incident," undated, www.nemsn.org/Articles/summary-tryptophan%20Fagan.htm (accessed June 3, 2005).

10. Lawrence Bachorik, "FDA Announces Withdrawal of Fenfluramine and Dexfenfluramine," HHS News, U.S. Department of Health and Human Services, September 15, 1997, www.fda.gov/bbs/topics/news/new00591.html (accessed November 22, 2005).

11. Marc W. Deitch (senior vice president at Wyeth-Ayherst Laboratories), "Letter to Health Care Professionals," December 1996, www.fda.gov/medwatch/safety/redux.htm (accessed November 22, 2005).

12. Paul G. Shekelle et al., "Efficacy and Safety of Ephedra and Ephedrine for Weight Loss and Athletic Performance," *Journal of the American Medical Association* 289 (2003): 1537–45.

13. Ibid.

14. Ibid.

15. Associated Press, "FDA Finalizes Ephedra Ban," February 6, 2004, www.cnn.com/2004/HEALH/diet.fitness/02/06/ephedra.ban.ap/ (accessed June 25, 2007).

16. Food and Drug Administration, "FDA Announces Rule Prohibiting Sale of Dietary Supplements Containing Ephedra Alkaloids Effective

April 12," April 12, 2004, www.fda.gov/bbs/topics/news/2004/new01050.html (accessed November 22, 2005).

17. Nathan Vardi, "Poison Pills: The Men and Money Pushing Dangerous Diet Supplements," *Forbes*, April 19, 2004, 79–86.

18. "Dangerous Supplements Still at Large," *Consumer Reports*, May 2004, 12–17.

19. M. Sovak et al., "Herbal Composition PC-SPES for Management of Prostate Cancer: Identification of Active Principles," *Journal of the National Cancer Institute* 94 (2002): 1275–81, and L. S. Marks et al., "PC-SPES: Herbal Formulation for Prostate Cancer," *Urology* 60 (2002): 369; both cited in Donald M. Marcus and Arthur P. Grollman, "Botanical Medicines: The Need for New Regulations," *New England Journal of Medicine* 347 (2002): 2073–76.

20. Marcus and Grollman, "Botanical Medicines."

21. Robert B. Saper et al., "Heavy Metal Content of Ayurvedic Herbal Medicine Products," *Journal of the American Medical Association* 292 (2004): 2868–79.

10

✚

How Can I Tell If the Evidence Is Any Good?

"Dr. Brown, you keep telling me all these bad things about alternative medicine, but the materials I read say that there is plenty of scientific evidence showing that alternative treatments work."

"Julie, that gets to the heart of the matter. If there is good evidence, based on double-blind, randomized, placebo controlled trials, that a treatment is safe and effective, then I am all for it. Too often, however, scientific claims are exaggerated. Let's look at the types of scientific evidence so you can read about these treatments more critically."

Caveat Emptor

In New York City, there are many individuals who legally sell things on the street. They are licensed by the city, and many set up shop on the same corner for years. For the most part, they sell merchandise that is inexpensive compared to what is sold in stores; often their wares are imitations of more expensive brands.

Sometimes, however, people without licenses, and without scruples, also sell things on the street. One sunny afternoon in July, a friend of mine was walking down the sidewalk when she noticed a crowd of people around a street vendor. The vendor was selling "personal stereos," the 1980s equivalent of iPods, for $10. Typically, personal stereos at the time were selling for at least $30 in stores.

Although this deal sounded too good to be true, this sidewalk entrepreneur was showing the customers the stereos, wrapped up and sealed in plastic bags. People who came by, including my friend, bought his whole stock rather quickly. When my friend got home, she discovered that the unit did not work. Most likely, an honest merchant had discarded these units. This enterprising young man had found them and used a device to seal them in plastic bags to enhance his credibility.

My friend had thought that she was saving a lot of money by buying something for a third of the usual price. Instead, she had just thrown away ten dollars. After this experience, she was more skeptical about buying things on the street, especially if the deal sounded too good to be true. After being swindled, she wanted vendors to prove that a device worked before she would buy it.

If you buy products because you believe false hype about them, you have been taken in, just as my friend was. As we have discussed, you have no legal protection in the world of alternative medicine. The rule is captured in the Latin phrase *caveat emptor*: "let the buyer beware."

I hope that this chapter will give you some of the tools you need to evaluate claims made by those who sell products promising health benefits. When someone tries to sell you a medical treatment, I want your reply to be "Prove it to me." In other words, what is the evidence that this helps? A doctor should be happy to answer that question, and so should any other person selling a treatment. But always remember that if something sounds too good to be true, it probably isn't true.

Understanding the Issues

"Dr. Brown, I am so glad that we're going to look at scientific evidence. I keep seeing advertisements that say studies show that natural remedies help people. Some of the products they advertise are the same ones that you've just told me are dangerous!"

"Julie, I won't pretend that I can teach you enough to analyze all of the evidence by yourself every time. But I do think that I can teach you enough to recognize some pitfalls when you look at the advertisements. To do that, let me start out by explaining how new knowledge is developed and communicated in the scientific community."

How Does New Information Get Out to the Scientific Community?

With rare exceptions, science does not grow by large leaps: it grows slowly and painstakingly, with one observation placed carefully atop another like bricks in a large wall. First, the bricks are put in without mortar to be sure that they are lined up properly. Then mortar is added, and they are locked in place. Sometimes a brick is out of line, perhaps because a preliminary observation turns out to be wrong or because a new discovery shows that things fit together differently than it appeared at first. Then a brick or even a whole portion of the wall has to be removed and reassembled.

What Is an "Abstract"?

When a brick is first discovered and the investigator thinks that *maybe* he knows where it might fit, he publishes what is called an abstract. An abstract is a short description, usually less than a page in length, of preliminary experiments. No mortar is allowed at this point. The purpose is to let other scientists know that this investigator may be onto something. On the other hand, he may not be onto anything at all, and the experiment may not even be reproducible. Many abstracts are published that turn out to be wrong, and they never lead to any progress. Every serious scientist knows that the information contained in an abstract is to be taken skeptically, because of the fact that it is *preliminary*.

What Is a "Paper"?

If the investigator confirms the information originally reported in an abstract or refutes it in a definitive way, he submits a journal article, known as a *paper*, for publication. The editor of the journal looks at the paper to determine whether the experiments were well designed and whether the information is important enough to be included in her journal. If she thinks that the paper may be worthwhile, she sends it out to two or more reviewers. Usually, the reviewers are other scientists working in the same field as the investigator. The reviewers make recommendations to the editor. Sometimes they recommend that the journal reject the paper, either because the experiments are not done properly or because the work is not unique. Alternatively, they can recommend that the journal publish the paper as submitted. Frequently, the reviewers will recommend that the paper be published but only after the investigator makes some changes, most commonly by doing additional experiments to confirm the ones he has already done. Because his fellow scientists review the work of the writer, a journal that uses this approach is called a "peer-reviewed journal."

As you can see, an abstract is a far cry from a paper. Basing any important decisions on an abstract, such as whether to take a supplement, is putting mortar in far too early.

When an investigator writes a paper, he submits it to the most prestigious journal he believes might accept it. Publishing in prestigious journals ensures that other scientists have access to his work. On a more selfish note, having papers in prestigious journals helps the investigator get tenure at his university. It gives him an advantage the next time he applies for a grant. It impresses other scientists at parties.

In any given field of medicine, there are only a handful of journals that are universally read. In most fields, this handful is between three and five. There are other journals, of course, but the other journals publish papers that are less important in their implications, less surprising in their results (perhaps because they confirm theories that are already established), or less definitive in their conclusions (perhaps because the experiments were not designed as well). This means that the universe of journals where the most important work is published is very small, containing fewer than a hundred publications in clinical medicine.

Is a Paper in a Good Journal the Final Word?

After a paper is published, it stimulates other scientists to try to add bricks to that area of the wall. The observations in the original paper will be reexamined and expanded in other experiments. Some scientists will try to disprove the results of the first paper. Eventually, there will be several papers on a given issue. Then another scientist will write a review paper, where she examines the results of all the experiments to date and tries to fit them together. It is only at this point that adding mortar is appropriate.

So in the hierarchy of publication, an abstract is strictly preliminary and is not to be accepted as fact under any circumstances. An initial paper is tentative and indicates that progress may have been made. Just how tentative an initial paper is depends on the quality of the work. Papers published in more prestigious journals are generally more significant than those published in obscure journals. But only after the initial paper is confirmed in other studies do we really *know* something scientifically.

Has Much Research Been Done on Alternative Medicine?

The National Institutes of Health (NIH) is the agency that gives out most government money for medical research in the United States. Within very broad guidelines, the NIH invites scientists to apply for money to do their research. A panel of other scientists then reviews the research proposals to assess how likely each proposal is to lead to a scientific advance. They assign a priority for funding to each proposal. The available money is then divided based on these priorities. It has always been possible to apply for funding of research in alternative treatments on the same standard as conventional approaches. If the evidence supporting alternative research is strong, it will receive funding.

In response to public pressure to spend more money studying alternative treatments, Congress established the Office of Alternative Medicine at the NIH in 1992. Unfortunately, the money has not led to results. In 1998, Marcia

Angell and Jerome Kassirer pointed out that of thirty grants awarded by this office in 1993, twenty-eight abstracts were produced, but only nine papers. Of these nine papers, five were published in journals not included in the Countway Library of Medicine, which contains 3,500 titles. Remember that as we discussed above, scientists try to publish their results in the most widely read journal they can. The most widely read journals make up a much shorter list than these 3,500 titles. The other four studies, published in journals that are in that list, did not reach conclusions about the efficacy of a single alternative treatment.[1]

I wish I could say that the situation has changed. Wallace Sampson looked at the status of investigations into alternative remedies in 2005. He reported that the NIH had spent $1.5 billion on research into complementary medicine from 1999 to that time and had failed to find any evidence that *any* of these treatments were effective. Sampson points out that these negative findings have not reduced the supplement industry's production of these products or the public's use of them. He notes that the industry often refuses to accept the studies that prove their products are ineffective.[2]

Should Tax Dollars Continue to Fund Studies on Alternative Medicine?

As Sampson discusses in his review, echinacea is an herbal treatment still being promoted for the treatment of viral upper-respiratory infections. Native Americans used it in the 1800s for conditions as different as sore gums and snakebite, and it continues to be used in folk medicine for all kinds of conditions. Its use developed when we had no understanding of the nature of disease and no theoretical framework for the study of potential treatments. Studies in recent years have shown that echinacea does stimulate immune-system cells, but only in the test tube. Unfortunately, this effect on cells in the test tube does not predict what happens in people. Until recently, the clinical studies on echinacea were inadequate to determine safety and efficacy. The study that occasioned Sampson's review of the funding of alternative medicine research was an excellent one that conclusively demonstrated that echinacea has *no benefit in people* with respect to upper-respiratory infections.[3]

Normally, as discussed above, NIH awards research funds on the basis of grant proposals. These proposals review the knowledge that exists on a given topic, the reasons (both theoretical and observational) that a scientist's ideas are likely to be true, and a proposed set of experiments to test the hypothesis. Sampson argues that the research on echinacea would never have been given tax dollars on that basis. There was no theoretical reason that echinacea would work and no convincing observational studies that suggested it would work. Why did we spend our tax dollars there rather than on something that had a reasonable chance for success? To study a so-called "remedy" because it is popular steals money from ideas that could save lives and relieve suffering.[4] Further, so-called complementary and alternative treatments have been able to apply for government grants through the usual mechanisms all along. Why give them their own office in the NIH?

Of course, the answer to that question is politics. Timothy Gorski, a physician who is president of the Dallas–Fort Worth Council Against Health Fraud, has summarized the formation of the Office of Alternative Medicine, which later became the National Center for Complementary and Alternative Medicine.[5] Senator Tom Harkin of Iowa pushed for the formation of the Office of Alternative Medicine (OAM) after he felt that bee pollen helped his hay fever symptoms.

After the OAM was formed, Gorski argues, Harkin pushed for governing members who were advocates of alternative medicine and discouraged critical scientific scrutiny of alternative treatments. Gorski documents that grants from this agency supported studies on psychic powers (referred to as "distant healing") and bizarre treatments for pancreatic cancer, including coffee enemas. Gorski also documents that most of the leaders of this agency are strong advocates of alternative therapies rather than individuals devoted to rigorous scientific examination of alternative claims.[6]

The bottom line, as both Sampson and Gorski point out, is that money spent testing implausible ideas and treatments would be better spent testing more promising approaches.

Types of Evidence for Alternative Treatments

"But the websites say that these treatments have been studied and shown to help," Julie assured me.

"I have spent a lot of time looking at various websites to examine the evidence cited for various products. It has been a rather disappointing experience. The 'proof' fell into several categories, which we will now discuss."

No Evidence at All

The first category is a failure to present any evidence at all. Many alternative websites claim that their products are superior to prescription drugs, claiming that these natural cures are more effective and less toxic. (As discussed in chapter 8, this claim is not logical. More potent medications, affecting our bodies more profoundly in positive ways, also have greater potential toxicity—greater potential to affect the body more profoundly in *negative* ways. The sharper the knife, the deeper it cuts, for good or for ill.) These websites attack conventional medicine and warn the reader how dangerous and bad it is. They may cite studies about the evils of the FDA or the toxicities of conventional medicine. They then assert that the alternative medicines that they market are better and give vague, theoretical reasons for it. Most do not, however, even pretend to present any evidence in the form of scientific literature to prove that their products are safe or effective.

In this same category is false presentation of evidence. The government recently settled a case against a seller of alternative remedies. The Federal Trade Commission alleged that while the company claimed that studies showed that its products reduced cholesterol, improved energy levels, and decreased symptoms in cancer patients, the studies referenced did not prove these benefits.[7]

The Testimonial

The second category of evidence is the testimonial. "My life was terrible, and I was dying of cancer. Then I found . . ." You can fill in the blank with whatever product is being sold. A testimonial is an individual's firsthand account of his or her personal experience. What is wrong with testimonials as scientific evidence?

Back in chapter 5, we learned that one of the difficulties with biological systems is *variability*. With a physics experiment, the results will be the same any day of the week. In the case of medical issues, the results are not so constant. No disease is 100 percent fatal, and no treatment is either 100 percent effective or 100 percent harmful. For example, for a terrible cancer, the two-year survival without treatment might be 2 percent. Perhaps with treatment, the two-year survival improves to 60 percent.

So with no treatment, two out of a hundred people will still be alive at the end of two years. If one of those two people tells you her story, that is a testimonial. I could use that testimonial to claim that no one should be treated at all, even though treatment would have improved their chances by a factor of 30. If instead of telling you only about the two who survived, I also tell you about the ninety-eight who died without treatment, I am giving you a fuller picture. Conversely, if my treatment is 60 percent effective and I cite only the experience of one of the survivors, that is also a testimonial. I need to tell you that 60 percent lived but also that 40 percent died.

The very nature of biology dictates statistics as the only way to determine your best option. Biological variability is the reason that nothing in medicine comes with a guarantee. It is one of the reasons that you go to the doctor and come away feeling that you have no idea what she said, because every statement has so many ifs, ands, and buts. This unavoidable uncertainty is the fertile ground in which the charlatan's confident, positive assertions grow and spread so quickly. It is also the reason that testimonials are inherently deceptive, because an individual testimonial cannot give you the whole story. Consider Megan:

Megan tried to remember exactly what she had said, but ten years had passed since the interview. She had been living in Salt Lake City at the time, and her chronic fatigue syndrome was the worst it had ever been. She was in bed most of the day. A friend suggested that she try a new mixture of herbs, vitamins, and minerals that a supplement company claimed would help. It took a few months, but she finally felt better. Both she and her husband wrote grateful letters to the company. Two weeks later, she found herself in front of a microphone at the local radio station being interviewed about her experience.

"Megan, tell our listeners about your life six months ago."

"It was terrible. I was in bed most of the time. I couldn't care for my husband or my children the way I wanted to. I didn't feel like doing anything."

"Had you been to your doctor?"

"Oh, yes. He tried to put me on antidepressants and an exercise program. I followed his advice, but the pills didn't help, and I was just too weak to exercise."

"Had you tried other supplements?"

"Anything I could get my hands on. But nothing seemed to help."

"How did you find CFS–Natural Cure?"

"A friend read about it in a magazine and suggested I try it."

"What happened after you started taking it?"

"Nothing happened at first. I took it for several months with no real change. Finally, though, I began to feel better. At first, I was able to be up for half a day, and now I can keep going all day long and into the night."

"What advice would you give our listeners with chronic fatigue syndrome?"

"I would encourage them to use CFS–Natural Cure. Even if it doesn't seem to help at first, keep taking it. Eventually you will feel a lot better."

She continued to take the supplement, but about two years later, her fatigue worsened again, and ever since she had continued to have periods of severe fatigue and periods when she felt reasonably well. She finally abandoned the supplement, since it was clear that it wasn't helping, with her ups and downs continuing to occur every year or two. Now she was desperate again and had gone onto the Internet to see if there was anything new.

After typing in "chronic fatigue," she had stumbled onto her own testimonial. There were the words that the com-

pany claimed she said in her radio interview a decade ago.

Since she had now lived with her disease another decade and read much more about it in the medical literature, she realized that good and bad times would come no matter what treatment plan she followed. She had mistaken the natural course of the disease for a response to the medicine. Her testimonial was helping this company promote a product that she now believed was nothing but a waste of money.

Now she was angry. She remembered the company owner, Trent Forchette-Boucher, and actually still had his telephone number.

"Sure, Megan, I remember you. I really appreciated your testimonial about our product. It continues to be a big help in aiding others with chronic fatigue syndrome."

"I want to withdraw my testimonial right now. I don't think your concoctions do doodle."

"Why do you say that, Megan?"

"My chronic fatigue is as bad as ever."

"Are you still taking CFS–Natural Cure?"

"No. I stopped taking it years ago when I realized that it didn't do anything."

"Well, maybe you just need to get back on it."

"Trent, you have to know by now that that's rubbish. Just get my testimonial off your website."

"Megan, I appreciate your concern and sincerity, but I'm not going to do that. Your testimonial is the best we have ever received, and you signed a contract agreeing that we could use your statements in perpetuity, forever. I would be happy to send you a free thirty-day supply of the newest version of CFS–Natural Cure."

"That won't be necessary."

As she slammed down the phone, she realized that there really was nothing she could do. If she went to a local tele-

vision or radio show, the most she would get would be a forty-second mention on the news. There was nothing she could do to take back her words. She glanced down at the web page and saw that its counter showed over a million hits that month alone.

As she continued to search the Internet, she did so with new insight. She ignored testimonials that she knew were misleading. She wanted to see scientific research, studies in which medicines were tested against placebos, studies that lasted longer than a month, studies that were done in reputable universities, studies that had been published in major medical journals. She realized that it would not help her to spend money on unproven treatments. If there was nothing new that was proven, she decided, she would participate in a proper research trial that might help her and help others. Maybe that would make up for the harm she had perpetuated.

Animal Research

The third category of research that is cited in support of alternative medicine is animal research. This category is a good example of the double standard often employed by advocates of alternative medicine.

"Mr. Jones, here is a prescription for a medication to lower your cholesterol."

"Dr. Brown, I really worry about the potential side effects of medications. What should I watch for with these pills?"

"I don't think you'll have any side effects. None of the rats they tried it on complained about any side effects."

"What do you mean?"

"It has only been tested in rats. It seemed to lower their cholesterol, and none of the rats had any problems that the investigators could see."

With that kind of approach, I would not last long as a cardiologist, yet people shell out millions of dollars when websites tout how well a product works in animals. Don't forget that any substance with the potential to affect you for good will have the potential to cause harm. Many drugs reach the level of testing in animals and seem to work. They go on to be tested in people and seem to work. And then, when the drugs are used in large numbers of people, we discover that they cause harm. It is unwise to take something into your body based on tests in animals alone.

Out-of-Date Research

A favorite trick of charlatans is the use of old studies that have already been disproved. The beauty of this approach from a sales standpoint is that you have a built-in set of arguments and studies you can cite to support your product.

The clearest example is chelation therapy. Chelation is the chemical removal of substances from the body. It was proposed in the 1950s that chelation might be helpful in the treatment of hardening of the arteries. The idea was that since blockages in the arteries often contain calcium, removal of calcium from the body might diminish these blockages. There were uncontrolled trials (no placebo group) that seemed to show benefit from chelation. There were small controlled trials that seemed to demonstrate benefit as well. But *large* controlled trials have since laid the matter to rest: chelation provides no benefit. In other words, the apparent benefit in the early uncontrolled studies turned out to be due to the placebo effect. But if I want to promote chelation, I can quote any of the old uncontrolled trials I want, and they will sound impressive.

Abstracts

Many of the studies cited on company websites are abstracts. Some of them are described as "presentations at meetings." This means that the information has not been published in a peer-reviewed journal. If the work had been published, the website would provide the reference to the *publication*. If the "presentation" is more than two years old and a paper is not referenced, that means that investigators never did enough research to come up with a credible paper.

Alternative medicine does not have a monopoly on using abstracts. Just last week, a pharmaceutical representative tried to show me an abstract about a drug. I told him to come back when he had a published paper. Taking any medication into your body based on an abstract is foolish.

Part of the Facts

A slanted presentation of evidence can also be used to suggest a product is effective. There may be several studies that favor a product and several that do not. If you hear only about the favorable studies, you do not have the whole picture. In the medical literature, the quickest way to get a full picture is to find a review article that looks at all of the available evidence and is published in a major journal. Major advances in medicine do not rely on a single study, since one study can be misleading. If there is strong evidence, there should be a review article somewhere.

Uncontrolled Trials

Uncontrolled trials—those with no placebo group—are not an effective way to assess how well a treatment works, as discussed in earlier chapters. Some websites contain published reports of uncontrolled studies. Often these reports will conclude by conceding that the results are preliminary and need to be confirmed in prospective, randomized, controlled trials. Sometimes they state that such trials are planned.

When you read a report like this, look at its date. In my experience, many of these reports are more than three years old. The failure to have a controlled trial reported within two years or so suggests that either the trial was not done or it was done and is not reported because the results were disappointing. Either way, until a placebo controlled trial is reported, no one can accurately assess the effectiveness of a treatment.

Small Trials

Many of the trials reported on the Internet are too small to be meaningful. With common health problems, a decent trial will have hundreds of participants. A definitive trial will have thousands of participants. There are a lot of preliminary reports with only ten patients.

Not Published in a Reputable Journal

The vast majority of studies reported on the Internet have not been published in reputable journals. Sometimes the documentation of the research will lead you to other websites, which means that the studies were never published anywhere except on the Internet. In other cases, the studies are published in journals that are devoted solely to alternative medicine. That is *not* a good sign. Research that shows important results will be published in a mainstream journal, whether the product is labeled alternative or conventional. The three major journals for general medical issues are the *New England Journal of Medicine*, the *Journal of the American Medical Association*, and *Lancet*. Research that is not as definitive but is still important will be published in one of the two or three leading journals in the relevant subspecialty of medicine.

Double-Blind, Randomized, Controlled Trials in Reputable Journals

Unfortunately, these are few and far between. The ones that have been conducted on alternative treatments have been disappointing. But if such a trial supports an alternative therapy, it must be accepted.

Largely because of the National Center for Complementary and Alternative Medicine, there are a growing number of double-blind, randomized, controlled trials that have been documented in reputable journals. So far, this has not been good news for alternative medicine.

Saw palmetto is a popular treatment for enlargement of the prostate gland. It had good *preliminary* data for efficacy, based on small trials, some of which were controlled. In 2002, a survey suggested that 2.5 million Americans were using this medication.[8] In February 2006, a larger controlled trial was published in the *New England Journal of Medicine*. The study looked at 225 men with prostate symptoms and followed them for a year. In this study, there was no difference in outcome between saw palmetto and placebo.[9] Therefore, this very popular supplement appears to be no more effective than a sugar pill.

Glucosamine and chondroitin are another pair of alternative therapies that have been broadly used, often in combination with each other. Preliminary studies seemed to show some benefit with these medications in the treatment of arthritis. Because of the limited effectiveness and potential toxicities of conventional medications, many doctors have recommended these medications, both in the United States and in Europe.

In February 2006, a study was published in the *New England Journal of Medicine* looking at whether these products had any benefit in arthritis of the knee. The study followed 1,583 patients for six months. Overall, the supplements did not produce any statistically significant improvement compared to placebo. There appeared to be some improvement in the group treated with a combination of glucosamine and chondroitin, but the improvement did not reach statistical significance. This led the investigators to look further at the results for patients with more severe symptoms. For this subgroup, the combination of the chondroitin and glucosamine did show significant improvement compared with placebo. This result has to be viewed as preliminary and requiring further study, since the trial was not designed to look specifically at those with worse symptoms.[10]

What does this trial allow us to conclude? An editorial in the same issue of the *New England Journal* reviewed this study as well as the previous medical literature about these compounds. The conclusion was that neither glucosamine hydrochloride nor chondroitin sulfate was better than placebo for knee pain but that the combination *might* have some value for those with severe pain.[11]

Do you have an attic or a storage closet—a crowded place where you store things that you will probably never use again but you just can't throw away? When I was growing up, we had an attic, filled with all sorts of things. It had the musty smell of dust and old clothes. When I was first old enough to climb up into the attic, it seemed to me like a trove of all sorts of treasures—old toys, favorite shirts, old appliances. As I shone a flashlight on a box that looked particularly enchanting, the edge of the light touched an object that looked like a long-lost toy. Unfortunately, when I turned the flashlight directly on the object, it was just a wadded-up piece of fabric. Looking in a dark room with a flashlight is like that. You may think that a pot of gold is at the edge of the light. But when you bring the full light to bear on the object, it turns out to be yellowed aluminum foil.

Good scientific research answers clearly the question we set out to answer but often raises other questions and other ideas, like half-seen objects at the edges of a flashlight beam. The glucosamine/chondroitin study set out to determine whether these drugs were effective in relieving pain in patients with osteoarthritis of the knee. In the group as a whole, the answer was that these products were no different from placebo. Analyzing various subgroups after the study is complete is like looking at the edge of the flashlight beam. We cannot conclude from this study that these drugs lessen severe knee pain. When a researcher does a study to address *directly* the value of glucosamine and chondroitin in severe pain, it may turn out that the combination does nothing at all, or it may turn out that the combination is helpful. Until *that* study is done, what will be found when the flashlight is directed at that corner remains a matter of speculation. Do not pay the price of a pot of gold for a product until you shine your flashlight directly on it and are sure it is what it appears to be.

How Do I Apply These Principles?

Assuming that you do not have a close friend with a Ph.D. in biostatistics, how can you evaluate the information you read on the Internet? The reality is that most people cannot do this alone.

I believe that it is wisest not to take anything into my body unless there is strong evidence that it is both safe and effective. The first thing to do when you have a health problem is to discuss it with your doctor and ask him or her what to do. If your doctor spontaneously suggests an alternative product, you should ask how well established it is that the product is safe and effective. Before taking the product, you should then read about it in one of the resources I review below. If it still looks good, it is reasonable to take it.

If your doctor does not spontaneously suggest an alternative product but you have decided that you want to consider taking one, you should ask your doctor about it. If your doctor says that available alternative treatments don't help, you should stop there. If your doctor recommends a treatment or indicates that one may be helpful, you should still read about it yourself before taking it.

I believe that the course of action outlined above is in your best interests. However, having been born longer ago than yesterday, I know that some people will not follow my advice. If you plan to take alternative treatments no matter what your doctor says, at least read about them in the resources below *and* at least inform your doctor that you are taking them.

Resources to Use in Evaluating Alternative Treatments

Alternative Medicine: The Christian Handbook, by Danul O'Mathuna and Walt Larimore, is a good resource with an overview of the evidence about specific alternative therapies.[12] Dr. Stephen Barrett's website www.quackwatch. com provides excellent, detailed, well-researched, and documented information about alternative therapies that have been disproved. *Consumer Reports* has also become a reasonably objective source of information about these treatments and typically has a couple of issues a year containing reviews of alternative therapies.

A Christian Perspective

Always remember that there are two sides to every story. As Proverbs 18:17 says, "The first to plead his case seems right, until another comes and examines him."

Even drugs that make it through the FDA approval process have arguments against them. It is important to remember that medicine is not perfect and that all of our decisions include uncertainty about how an individual will respond to a treatment.

When I get permission from a patient to do a surgical procedure, I try to be sure that the patient understands the risks, benefits, and alternatives to the procedure. The risks are the bad things that might happen and some estimate as to how likely they are to occur. The benefits are the good things that we hope will happen and how likely they are to occur. The alternatives include both what is likely to happen if we do nothing and what is likely to happen if we use medication or a different procedure instead of the one I am proposing.

These same issues—risks, benefits, and alternatives—should be considered for every medical therapy, whether conventional or alternative. Asking about all three with any treatment can help you get both sides of the story.

Another website that provides a lot of information that is updated fairly often is presented by the Mayo Foundation for Medical Education and Research. However, as we will see, the information it provides has a bias in favor of alternative medicine. The website, www.mayoclinic.com, has a directory of both prescription drugs and supplements.[13]

When you type in the name of a prescription medicine in the search field of the Mayo site, the description you get is filled with warnings about potential side effects and potential dangerous adverse effects. You do not find much of a description of the good things the drug does or the evidence that it saves lives in certain circumstances. In the case of one drug I looked up, there were four sentences about beneficial effects and three pages of warnings.

If instead you type in the name of a supplement, you get information about the background of the product, a limited description of the evidence for its use, and a list of potential uses with a letter grade for each indicating to what extent scientific evidence supports the use of the product. There is some information about potential side effects and adverse effects to the extent that they are known.

There has been a lot of criticism of grade inflation in schools, where many children get undeserved As when they should be getting Bs and Cs. The grade inflation on this website is a lot worse than in today's schools.

Even the drugs and indications that get an A have major qualifications in the descriptions, such as that studies have given conflicting results, or that the studies are not of very good quality, or that more studies are needed to determine safety and effectiveness. I certainly would not give an A to a drug whose evidence is that weak.

However, I do applaud the website for providing much more complete information about these products than is available most places and for summarizing a lot of complicated information. If you choose to take a supplement, read the description on the Mayo website. If the product gets less than an A, I would urge you to stay away from it.

The difference in the nature of information provided for conventional and alternative products is likely due to the source of the information, rather than by design on the part of the Mayo Clinic Foundation. The website indicates that the information about conventional drugs is provided by Micromedex and the information about alternative products is provided by the Natural Standard Research Collaboration. Since different sources are used for the two sets of products, the information is not presented in the same way.

If you take a supplement, as discussed in chapter 9, you have no assurance that the supplement you buy contains what the label tells you. Another website, www.consumerlab.com, reports on the analysis of various alternative products so you can find out which brands are likely to contain what their manufacturers claim.

A Worldview Perspective

Why don't doctors come out more forcefully against alternative treatments? One of the reasons is that given their scientific orientation, doctors are reluctant to say that a treatment does *not* work until it has been tested and proved ineffective.

The problem with this scientific conservatism is that it allows alternative medicine companies to assume that their products are safe and effective and requires scientists to prove that they are not. This faulty assumption underlies the terrible harm that has been caused by the change in U.S. law in 1994. Modern medicine has been successful because it starts with the assumption that new treatments are ineffective and dangerous and makes them prove themselves in an uphill battle. Conventional medicine needs to refuse to allow alternative medicine to frame the issue. We must insist that any treatment is *ineffective* until proved otherwise.

Summary

Now that you know more about the scientific literature, you are better able to study both conventional and alternative treatments and discuss them with your doctor. Quite a few nonscientific arguments are used to support alternative medicine, and we will examine these in chapter 11.

Notes

1. Marcia Angell and Jerome P. Kassirer, "Alternative Medicine: The Risks of Untested and Unregulated Remedies," *New England Journal of Medicine* 339 (1998): 839–41.

2. Wallace Sampson, "Studying Herbal Remedies," *New England Journal of Medicine* 353 (2005): 337–39.

3. Ronald B. Turner et al., "An Evaluation of Echinacea angustifolia in Experimental Rhinovirus Infections," *New England Journal of Medicine* 353 (2005): 341–48.

4. Sampson, "Studying Herbal Remedies."

5. Timothy N. Gorski, "A Written Response to the Statement of the Honorable Dan Burton (R-IN), Chairman, House Committee on Government Reform," *U.S. Special Committee on Aging, Hearing on Swindlers, Hucksters, and Snake Oil Salesmen: The Hype and Hope of Marketing Anti-aging Products to Seniors*, September 10, 2001, available at www.quackwatch.org/01QuackeryRelatedTopics/Hearing/gorski2.html (accessed June 17, 2006).

6. Ibid.

7. William Blumenthal, Karen Muoio, and Michael Ostheimer (Federal Trade Commission), "Complaint for Permanent Injunction and Other Equitable Relief," U.S. District Court, Southern District of Florida, Federal Trade Commission, plaintiff, v. Garden of Life, Inc., and Jordan S. Rubin, defendant, 12–13, www.ftc.gov/os/caselist/gardenoflife/GardenofLifecomplaint.pdf (accessed June 17, 2006).

8. P. M. Barnes et al., "Complementary and Alternative Medicine Usage among Adults: United States," *Advance Data* 343 (2004): 1–19, cited in Stephen Bent et al., "Saw Palmetto for Benign Prostatic Hyperplasia," *New England Journal of Medicine* 354 (2006): 557–66.

9. Bent et al., "Saw Palmetto."

10. Daniel O. Clegg et al., "Glucosamine, Chondroitin Sulfate, and the Two in Combination for Painful Knee Osteoarthritis," *New England Journal of Medicine* 354 (2006): 795–808.

11. Marc C. Hochberg, "Nutritional Supplements for Knee Osteoarthritis: Still No Resolution," *New England Journal of Medicine* 354 (2006): 858–60.

12. Danul O'Mathuna and Walt Larimore, *Alternative Medicine: The Christian Handbook* (Grand Rapids: Zondervan, 2001).

13. The conventional-drug example of product information here is regarding Lipitor (atorvastatin), www.mayoclinic.com/health/drug-information/DR203635 (accessed June 20, 2006). The alternative-drug examples were saw palmetto, www.mayoclinic.com/health/saw-palmetto/NS_patient-sawpalmetto, and glucosamine, www.mayoclinic.com/health/glucosamine/NS_patient-glucosamine (both accessed June 20, 2006).

11

✚

What about Other Claims Made by Some Alternative Practitioners?

"I hate to bother you with this, Dr. Brown," Julie went on, "but there are still ideas about alternative medicine that I need to discuss with you. Some of them sound silly, perhaps because they are silly, but I would feel better if we talked about them. What about the claims about alternative medicine that have nothing to do with research?"

"Let's look at some of those."

Do Doctors and Drug Companies Conspire to Hide the Truth?

The very concept that a conspiracy involving millions of people could last more than a few seconds is frighteningly naive. Most people go into medical research dreaming of finding a cure for cancer, helping people, and perhaps winning a Nobel Prize. In addition, they have diseases of their own and families of their own. Investigators are often attracted to studying a particular disease because of a friend or family member with that condition. Why would they want to hide breakthroughs when this would hurt themselves and their own family?

The motive ascribed to doctors and drug companies for hiding these wonderful discoveries is that if the disease were cured, company profits would plummet. Therefore, the argument continues, doctors protect their livelihood by hiding the cures.

A research laboratory includes not only the lead investigator but also technicians, junior investigators, graduate students, undergraduate students, and postdoctoral fellows, all of whom are deeply involved in the process of discovery. When research reaches beyond the test tube to the level of clinical studies, hundreds of people are typically involved. So if this stadium full of people discovers something so grand, a cure so complete, that it will markedly reduce the need for doctors and drug companies, do you really think that they all will keep quiet? Any of them could easily get a job at another company who would develop the product or could readily go to the press or the U.S. Congress with the news, even if their primary employer tried to suppress it. With so many people involved, secrecy would be impossible.

Much of the research that breaks important ground is done in the academic setting. Investigators in that setting typically do not make money from drug sales but instead get money through the competitive funding of grants to do research. Most funding for research in universities is from government grants. Even in cases where a university investigator is partially funded by a grant from industry, the announcement of a great breakthrough would ensure success in academics. These scientists have no vested interest in hiding positive results. Positive results ensure that they can get their next grant, or get tenure, or become famous. Why would they hide good news? Ironically, to make such discoveries, these researchers had to be looking for cures in the first place. How do they decide what to suppress? Do they only suppress the ones that work too well?

As unrealistic as these conspiracy theories are, their corollary is even more absurd. The alternative medicine industry claims that while doctors are hiding these cures, the alternative industry has found them and is now promoting them through its advertising on the Internet. They must use the Internet because the news media are in on the conspiracy and do not want to report the truth that hundreds of people are being cured of cancer without surgery. Now if you can believe that the news media would not be interested in such a story, with its scandal, intrigue, and popular appeal, you must not have much exposure to the media.

On a personal note, I find it offensive that after making so many sacrifices to help people, I would be accused of hiding helpful treatments. If something is out there that will help my patients, I don't care where it came from or who will profit from it: I want it for my patients. That includes alternative treatments and treatments that represent a change from conventional medical viewpoints.

From a medical perspective, the idea of easy cures is an overly optimistic view of medical advances. Actual *cures* are few and far between. Medicine usually is only a way to treat and control disease.

From a historical perspective, I have to ask, "Where's the beef?" In numerous cases drug companies have been accused of covering up *adverse* effects of medications; some of these cases have been discussed in this book. Invariably, these result in lawsuits. There has never been a documented case where a drug company has covered up *beneficial* effects of a medication. If there were such a widespread conspiracy, there should have been all kinds of lawsuits by now, and whoever uncovers the conspiracy will be rich for life.

Part of the push for this theory occurs when an alternative medicine advocate is arrested for fraud. "There, you see! There *is* a conspiracy. That's why I was fined a million dollars—*they* arrested me." To believe this whopper, you have to believe that even though the person is innocent, a jury was convinced that she broke the law. Since these are criminal trials, the jury must be convinced in open court, where each side gets to present its own evidence, that beyond a reasonable doubt the products are ineffective. Even a reasonable doubt would force them to issue a not-guilty verdict. A criminal conviction or settlement is, in reality, about as close to proof of fraud as the public is ever likely to get without researching the issues themselves.

Doesn't Conventional Medicine Just Treat Symptoms?

Ever hear of the Human Genome Project? Massive amounts of money and resources were invested in deciphering the entire DNA code, in the hope that this will allow us to know what genes cause various diseases as well as how they do it. This project is a huge example, but the principle is general: I have never been to a medical lecture or read a medical journal article about any health problem that does not at least attempt to address the question of *cause*.

Much of what we do in medicine is directed at causes before symptoms even occur. For example, we know that blockages in the arteries are caused by high blood pressure and high cholesterol, so we use medicines to control these *causes*. "But what causes high blood pressure and high cholesterol?" Many of our therapies were developed as investigators asked that question. For example, high cholesterol is often caused by overproduction of cholesterol by an enzyme in the body called HMGCoA reductase, so we have learned to use drugs that inhibit this enzyme. "Well, what causes the enzyme to be overactive?" That question is under investigation at the level of the genes involved.

Does alternative medicine really treat causes? If you keep reading the advertisements where that assertion is made, you do not find a detailed scientific explanation about how "natural" medicines work. Instead, there is a vague assertion that the alternative treatment "restores balance" (remember the ancient Greeks) or that alternative treatment "harnesses the body's natural healing mechanisms." Of course, all medical treatments "harness the body's natural healing mechanisms." Even surgery that removes or repairs broken parts relies on the body to heal the wounds, so this claim is far from unique to alternative medicine.

To prove that a treatment gets at the cause, you must first determine what the cause is, at the level of molecules. Then you must show what your treatment does at the molecular level to reverse that cause. I have yet to see that level of knowledge about an alternative product.

But I Feel Better When I Take This Pill!

This argument is based on the idea that we can use our own experience to determine whether a treatment works or not. This gets to the concept introduced in chapter 7:

All of us are subject to bias. That includes me. It includes you. If you're not so sure about this, please reread chapter 7. Can you admit that maybe, just maybe, you could be subject to the placebo effect yourself? If not, can you at least admit that you might have gotten better on your own and the relationship to the medicine could be just a coincidence?

Individual experience is inherently subjective and every bit as misleading as any other testimonial. For us to know whether a treatment helps, it must be subjected to proper, placebo controlled testing.

How Can a Product That Has Been Used for Thousands of Years Not Be Effective?

Several years ago, it was discovered that a particular physician had a high rate of complications with his surgery. As the chairman of the committee that had investigated these complications presented his findings to the medical executive committee, he not only reported a high rate of complications but also noted that the complications were due to carelessness and incompetence. Another physician found the committee's findings hard to believe.

"How can this be? He has twenty years of experience."

"He doesn't have twenty years of experience," came the wise retort. "He has had the same one year of experience twenty times."

If I do not learn from my experience by asking the right questions, seeing my mistakes, and carefully testing new approaches, then I do not grow. I am the same way I was before I had any experience at all. This doctor was like that. He did not recognize, learn from, or even remember his complications. When another doctor tried to suggest that another approach might have been more effective, he would become angry and argumentative. He refused to learn from his mistakes.

The fact that an Eastern culture has used a certain herb for thousands of years means no more than the fact that Western culture used bleeding as a treatment for thousands of years. Scientific progress did not start until tradition was abandoned as a way of determining truth and observation took its place.

Do not use a treatment just because it is old. There were plenty of wrong ideas in the ancient world, both in the East and in the West. I do not want to give up modern conveniences, either technological or medical, to replace them with the life of the ancients.

Aren't Supplements Better at Maintaining Health, While Conventional Medicine Is Better for Injuries?

What is the difference between maintaining health and treating injuries? *There is no difference.* A knife between the ribs is obviously a physical problem. But the gradual buildup of blockages in your arteries is also a physical problem. So is the mutation that produces a cancer cell. Determining what works for prevention is the same process as determining what works for treatment. The process starts with observations, moves to hypotheses, then concludes with double-blind, randomized, placebo controlled trials.

The medical literature discusses preventive medicine at least as much as treatment of disease and trauma. Some approaches to prevention have worked, and others have not. If you want to know how to prevent disease, you need to study prevention the same way you study treatment.

Aren't Conventional Medications Dangerous?

What is safer, a treatment containing a single ingredient that has been extensively studied with the risks well defined or a pill containing thirty-seven ingredients, none of which has been studied enough for us to know the risks? All drugs have risks, and the risks are directly related to the potency of the drug: more potent drugs have more risks. But health problems are dangerous, too. The question is which do you prefer: (1) the disease untreated, (2) the disease treated with an extensively studied treatment shown to help and

A Christian Perspective

Diets "Based on the Bible"

Some alternative advocates claim that following the diets eaten on earth before Noah's flood will lead to longevity. They note the extraordinarily long lives reported for early biblical patriarchs and theorize that there was something about their diet that led to their longevity.

If there is some secret biblical diet that leads to longevity, it is hard to understand why it was not discovered until the twentieth or twenty-first century. Of course, the patriarchs lived before the dietary laws were given to Moses, so it is also hard to understand why such secrets were not incorporated in the instructions God gave his people or, if they were, why the Israelites who followed these laws did not have the same longevity as the patriarchs.

That a biblical diet leads to longevity has an even greater hurdle in the New Testament. Jesus says in Mark 7 that what a person takes into his body does not make him unrighteousness but that what matters is what comes out. He explains that what a person takes in through the mouth goes to the stomach and then is eliminated. "Thus he declared all food clean" (Mark 7:19).

Medically, this statement means that food stays outside the body, in the cavity that begins at the mouth and ends at the other end. Whatever actually enters the body, leaving this cavity, is filtered by the lining of the intestine. Only what the body chooses is absorbed into the bloodstream. The remainder leaves the body as waste.

So, Jesus says, food does not make us unrighteous. It is what comes out from our heart that shows our unrighteousness. He lists various sins that come out of us, beginning with evil thoughts.

When Christianity started, it was exclusively a Jewish religion, and the early believers assumed that it was not open to Gentiles. In Acts 10–11, Peter is taught by God that Gentiles are also welcome to worship Jesus. God teaches him this through a dream where he is told that God has made unclean animals clean. In other words, God is eliminating the Jewish legal restrictions on various foods. As recounted in Acts 15, the Jewish leaders had a meeting to decide whether the laws of Moses should be applied to the Gentiles. They concluded that the Gentiles should be instructed to abstain only from "things contaminated by idols and from fornication and from what is strangled and from blood" (Acts 15:20). To put Christians back under other dietary restrictions is not easily reconciled with the teaching of the book of Acts.

I am not saying that diet does not matter. We know that what we eat affects our risk for heart disease, cancers, and digestive problems. What I am saying is that to claim divine sanction for a particular diet is difficult to reconcile with the whole of scripture.

Aren't Testimonials a Biblical Way to Determine Truth?

Some Christians have taught that testimonials are an acceptable way to determine truth with respect to "natural cures." They base their argument on the law of Moses. Jesus cites this law during a discussion with the Pharisees. The Pharisees are arguing that his claims of deity are not true because he makes the claims about himself. Jesus responds in John 8:14–18:

> Even if I testify about Myself, My testimony is true, for I know where I came from and where I am going; but you do not know where I come from or where I am going. You judge according to the flesh; I am not judging anyone. But even if I do judge, My judgment is true; for I am not alone in it, but I and the Father who sent Me. Even in your law it has been written that the testimony of two men is true. I am He who testifies about Myself, and the Father Who sent Me testifies about Me.

The legal principle that Jesus talks about is in Deuteronomy 17:6, which states that when someone is charged with a capital crime, they are not to be put to death on the testimony of one witness but there must be at least two or three witnesses.

In claiming that his witness is true, Jesus invokes his personal knowledge of the issues. He also invokes the corroboration of God the Father. How did the Father bear witness of Jesus to the Pharisees? He did not appear to this group of Pharisees and talk to them audibly. Instead, the Father bore witness of Jesus through the scriptures, his direct revelation to his people. Jesus was pointing the Pharisees to the Bible. A few chapters earlier, in John 5:39, he points out to them, "You search the Scriptures, because you think that in them you have eternal life; it is these that testify about Me. . . ."

So in discussing the use of testimony, Jesus invokes the importance of both personal knowledge and validation by objective information. The concept of testimony in the law does not mean that anything that two people agree about is true, no matter what evidence exists to the contrary. If that were the case, any heresy that two people agreed about would be established as sound doctrine.

In other words, even though having two witnesses may be necessary to establish truth, it is not sufficient to establish truth. Harry's story provides a good example of the problem with using testimony alone to establish the facts.

Harry stood before the group and began to share his story.

"My life was difficult. I was in a marriage that was empty. My wife wanted me to go for counseling, but I didn't see the point. One day I met Katherine. She was everything I had ever wanted. She was beautiful, elegant, and engaging. Soon I found myself at her apartment almost every night, and I finally divorced my wife. Now Katherine and I are living together. I still have a good relationship with my children. Katherine is the best thing that ever happened to me: without our adulterous relationship, I would still be in a dead-end marriage."

What is wrong with Harry's testimonial? Should we listen to him and adopt his worldview? Why not?

The first problem with Harry's testimonial is that it *contradicts God's revelation in scripture*. The Bible is quite clear that adultery is wrong. On this basis alone, it does not matter how many people claim that adultery is a good thing; as a Christian who accepts the authority of God's revelation, I will reject this claim. In the same way, health claims need to be compared to God's revelation in both scripture and the world of nature, which is where double-blind, randomized, controlled trials come in. It does not matter how many people claim that a treatment has helped them, until you know what happened to the placebo group and thereby have objective information to validate or invalidate a testimonial.

This issue gets to the second problem with Harry's testimonial. One testimonial *never* contains the whole story. In this example, the story is incomplete until you talk with Harry's ex-wife and their children, as well as considering what might have happened if Harry had gone for marriage counseling as his wife requested. Longer-term follow-up is also important. If he is like a lot of men, he will eventually leave Katherine also and end up with a third partner, and then Katherine will, perhaps, not be so happy anymore.

Testimonials are inherently subjective and incomplete. You need a chance to cross-examine Harry and to question the others who are involved. You need to take a skeptical view of claims like his or any other claims about truth. Again, "The first to plead his case seems right, until another comes and examines him" (Prov. 18:17).

The idea that two witnesses are *sufficient* to establish truth is a destructive one. All claims must be held up to the light of God's revelation. As Romans 3:4 says, "Rather, let God be found true, and every man be found a liar." Not only are two witnesses not sufficient to establish truth, even if every person on the planet claimed something that contradicts God's revelation, it would still not be true.

To apply this concept explicitly to health care: because of our human frailty, testimonials cannot provide meaningful personal knowledge. Even though they may provide clues that merit investigation, scientific study to assess objective truth is imperative to evaluate any proposed treatments.

But They Appear on Christian Television, on Christian Radio, and in Christian Magazines

I hope that someday this will mean something, but this means nothing at present. Fuzzy thinking about issues of truth has led to a wide acceptance of ineffective therapies in the Christian community. I hope information and concerns like those presented in this book will lead to higher standards in what is accepted as advertising and who is invited to appear in the Christian media.

The typical writer of an infomercial about getting rich in real estate would not be invited to appear on a Christian talk show, but somehow anyone who claims to have an easy, "natural" way to greater health is welcomed with open arms. Some of these individuals are physicians. Almost all are selling something. Often they claim that scientific evidence supports their claims. Unfortunately, their claims are generally unrealistic and far outside established medical fact. Why are they invited to be on television shows that generally focus on spiritual health? Why are they not treated with skepticism?

One of my motivations for writing this book was the fact that Christians, who ought to be more skeptical than others, are instead often the most willing to believe whatever they hear. I hope and pray that this will stop. Christians should be the most reluctant to take anything into their body that does not have strong evidence of safety and efficacy, and we should be the most enthusiastic in accepting help when an approach is proved to be helpful.

to have only small risks, or (3) the disease treated with a product that has not been adequately studied to determine whether it is safe or effective?

All medications, natural and alternative, are dangerous. They should be avoided, but not at *all* costs. They should be avoided unless the benefits exceed the risks. As discussed in chapter 9, the risks of supplements are at least as great as the risks of conventional medicine.

This deception is one of the most serious I have discussed. Many patients, like Julie, are afraid to take life-saving medications because of exaggeration of the risks of conventional medications and an underestimation of the risks of disease without medications. Doctors end up having to dispel a lot of false notions in order to save lives. Sometimes the deceptions are so strong that we are unable to do so, and people die as a result. This is probably the most damaging legacy of the alternative medicine industry.

Are the Purveyors of Alternative Medicine All Evil?

I guess it may sound as if I think so, but I really don't, anymore than I think all medical doctors are evil. There are certainly purveyors of alternative medicine who are evil and who engage in deliberately deceptive advertising practices. However, there is a much larger group of individuals who believe in these products. Unfortunately, their belief does not render their treatments safe or effective. Some of them believe in the products because of testimonials of themselves or people they know. Some believe in them because the concept of "natural healing" is appealing to them philosophically. Some of them have accepted the weak scientific evidence for some of the products without adequate criticism. All of them, like all of us, are subject to bias.

One of my greatest hopes for this book is that it will encourage the honest individuals in the alternative industry to step back, examine the facts, and recognize that their industry is doing a lot of harm (mostly by causing people to resist lifesaving therapies) and not doing much good. Many individuals in the alternative industry are aging and will reach a point when, despite taking all the substances that are supposed to prevent disease, they themselves face a health crisis. Perhaps you are in that category. At that point, many of them will recognize that the unrealistic claims that they have heard are just that: unrealistic.

Doesn't Alternative Medicine Focus on the Whole Person While Conventional Medicine Addresses Only Disease?

I certainly hope conventional medicine does not focus just on disease. I, for one, was taught in medical school to look at the whole person. Much of our curriculum during the transition from basic science to the bedside focused on the nonphysical aspects of disease. I try to look at my patients as whole people and to consider nonphysical aspects of their lives that play a role in their illness and may play a role in their healing.

The attraction of this accusation is the dissatisfaction that many of us feel in interacting with our doctors. We feel that they don't listen or don't understand our situation. We should certainly try to find a doctor who listens and cares about us. However, the most important attribute of a caregiver is whether what they offer can help us.

If I need surgery, I would prefer a good surgeon with no bedside manner to a bad surgeon with good bedside manner. If I have a choice, a good surgeon with good bedside manner is even better. But too often, alternative practitioners are approaching your health problems with unproved treatments. No matter how lovingly administered, the use of unproven treatments is a poor choice.

But Doctors Recommend This Treatment.

I wish that this meant more. Unfortunately, there are both dishonest and biased medical doctors who do not practice medicine based on scientific evidence.

One of the purposes of this book is to encourage you to take charge of your health care by insisting on understanding the rationale behind your treatment. If your doctor recommends a treatment that is outside conventional medicine, he or she needs to explain the evidence behind it. Be wary when your doctor says things like "This is not mainstream medicine, but I have found that it works. I am ahead of a lot of medical doctors in the treatment of your problems."

If you hear things like that, run, do not walk, to the nearest exit. Statements like these show bias, subjectivity, and a lack of objective evidence. If a doctor who bases her practice on *evidence* is doing something new, she will tell you, "This is a new treatment. The latest studies show that it reduces your risk of death and improves your chances for a full recovery."

Summary

"Does that answer your questions, Julie?"

"I think so, Dr. Brown. If I understand you, you're saying that all that really matters is whether a treatment has been properly studied. If it has not been proven, we should stay away from it. Despite all the hype, most alternative therapies are not proven. And despite our desire to be cured by conventional medicines, all of these involve risks, too. It's just that we know the risks of conventional medicines and too often we don't know the risks of alternative medicines."

"Julie, you have the idea. I want to guide you through this difficult journey. Please bring in your questions and any ideas that you hear about cardiac health. We will discuss them together. If you bring in an idea from alternative medicine that is valid, I will be happy to say so. If the ideas are unproven, I will tell you that also. My first and only concern is to do all I can to help you live as long as you can and as well as you can."

PART **4**

✚

THE
PATIENT

12

✚

How Can I Deal with My Illness?

"Dr. Brown, your counsel on dealing with my illness and navigating the medical maze means a lot to me. I want your help to make it through this as well as I can. My problem now is that even though I understand the science, I am terrified of my heart problem. It is really eating my lunch."

"Well then, Julie, let's talk about how to deal with health problems like yours on a personal, emotional level."

When Health Problems Eat Your Lunch

What gets under your skin? What commandeers your emotions, destroys your ability to concentrate, and monopolizes your thoughts? For Indiana Jones, it was snakes. For many of us, it is health problems in ourselves or in a loved one.

I know what you're going through. There are others who face the same struggles you do. Let's consider some of their stories.

Carrie Compton is a stay-at-home mom who rides her exercise bicycle faithfully three times a week but has never lost the weight she gained with her third child. All her brothers and sisters have high blood pressure. Most of her family started on blood pressure medications in their thirties, but she is now forty-two and still is not on medicine. In the last few months, Carrie has checked her blood pressure at the machine in the grocery store at least once a week. The numbers are always in the 150s over the 80s. The goal is to have the top number less than 140.

Summer sunlight from the window shines on her brown hair, accentuating her soft features and casting shadows across the furrows in her brow. She is obviously anxious and fearful about her blood pressure.

"Dr. Brown, I don't want to start on medicine, but I don't want to have a stroke either."

After discussing the options, we choose a blood pressure medication that seems right for her. She is to return in a week so we can see how the medicine is working.

Two days later, my nurse asks to talk with me between patients.

"Carrie Compton called. She says that ever since you started her on that blood pressure pill, she has felt jittery and anxious. I tried to tell her that those symptoms should not be from the medicine and that she should try to stick with it, but she said she doesn't want to take it anymore."

"That's fine. Let's just put her on a different medicine and check her blood pressure in a week."

Remember the "nocebo" effect, where a person is firmly convinced that a negative symptom they experience is related to a medication, even though the medicine has nothing to do with it. The medicine I had chosen for Carrie does not cause anxiety. Nonetheless, she was firmly convinced that it did. At this point, it was simplest just to change medications.

Two days later, Carried called back, convinced that the second medicine was also making her jittery and anxious. After she changed to a third medicine, the same thing happened. I had her come in for an office visit.

"Carrie, you're pretty upset about having high blood pressure, aren't you?"

"Yes, Dr. Brown. A lot of people in my family had high blood pressure and eventually died of strokes. Every time I think about my high blood pressure, I am afraid the same thing will happen to me."

"You know, Carrie, a lot of people who develop high blood pressure or high cholesterol feel as if someone has told them how they are going to die. Is that how you feel?"

"It sure is. I can't stop thinking about it. Up until now, I never thought much about the fact that I will die someday. Now I worry about my children and my husband. I wonder what it will feel like one day to be in the hospital with a stroke."

"Carrie, what you are experiencing is normal. Many people with a new health problem go through a period of adjustment, feeling anxious, upset, and frightened. Many people who have a heart attack actually develop depression and need to go on antidepressant medication, most of them for about a year.

"Carrie, none of the three medicines you have tried for blood pressure has anxiety as a recognized side effect. Do you think maybe you are jittery and anxious about having high blood pressure and that maybe these symptoms are not from the medicines at all?"

"I don't know, Dr. Brown. The anxiety sure seemed to start when I started the medicine."

"Of course it did. Taking the medicine accentuated the fact that you have high blood pressure. Carrie, I always say that any medicine *can* do anything to any given individual. But to have the same unrecognized side effect from three different medications does not make any scientific sense."

"I guess you're probably right, Dr. Brown. I guess I am just really upset about having high blood pressure. What should we do?"

As I explained to Carrie, fear and anxiety are common reactions for people facing a new illness. A new health problem, especially for someone who has been healthy, can be hard to swallow. Like many other stresses in life, health issues can eat your lunch.

The first step to dealing with our anxiety is to recognize it. After going through three different medicines, Carrie was able to step back and see that her reactions did not make sense. How could *all* of these medications make her anxious? Her perception must not be accurate. Depression and anxiety do that: they distort what we see. This distortion makes it hard to separate our emotions from the facts.

Once we recognize our fear, we need to analyze the facts as objectively as possible. In Carrie's case, she realized that having high blood pressure does not really tell her how she will die or when she will die. Instead, knowing that she has high blood pressure gave us an opportunity to make her live longer and *avoid* a stroke. Avoiding the medicines would have been like burying her head in the sand, trying to deny the problem. Instead, she needed to use medication to *solve* the problem.

When Health Problems Eat Your Supper, Too

Several years ago, a patient of mine with Alzheimer's disease, Mr. James Mason, had to have his arm amputated. Before the amputation, he was always quiet and cooperative, even though he could no longer talk and had no memory of what had happened even a few minutes before. After the amputation, several times a day he would suddenly become agitated, swinging his stump around and screaming until he was exhausted. Although he couldn't communicate verbally, I believe that every time he happened to look down, he rediscovered that his arm was gone. The horror he felt every time was just as bad as the first time, since there was no memory and therefore no passage of time to heal this open psychological wound.

Sometimes even after we recognize a fear and analyze the facts, the anxiety does not go away. We forget about it for a few minutes or a few hours, but then we glance over and see it, like Mr. Mason's stump. The fear jumps up and grabs us, and holds our head under the icy water of terror, until we are sure we will drown.

For some of us, this kind of terror is aroused by health problems. Some people deal with a terminal illness with easy grace but are gripped with terror by financial problems. Others have this kind of anxiety about legal problems or disrupted family relationships. But sooner or later, most of us will have some experience that makes us feel this way.

Joann Peyton's daughter, Phyllis, has leukemia. Joann is always preoccupied about Phyllis and spends a great deal of time caring for her. Joann has aged ten years in the past two. With her daughter's death now imminent, she does not know how she will cope with the loss, even though she knows her daughter's quality of life is now poor.

Emma Burton is sixty-five years old and is raising her grandson, Timothy. Her adopted daughter Tina is addicted to drugs and has been in and out of prison several times. Because Tina was not caring for Timothy properly, Emma got legal custody. The boy has been diagnosed with attention deficit disorder and requires constant supervision. When Emma had to go into the hospital for testing, she was very worried about being sure he had proper care. She does not know who will care for him if something happens to her.

Michael Phillips is a patient of mine who developed high blood pressure at the age of fifty. His prognosis for a normal lifespan was excellent. Aside from the inconvenience of taking medication regularly, there was no need for a change in his active, healthy lifestyle. Even though he knew this intellectually, for the first two years after his diagnosis he could not deal with his anxiety. He was afraid to go to work. He was afraid to go to sleep. He was afraid to be alone. He stayed out of work for months until he could get a grip on his emotions. A benign health problem did great harm to his life for a long time.

I wish I could give you an easy answer to the stress associated with problems like these, but I don't have one. I *can* tell you about some approaches that have helped other people.

After we recognize the fear and analyze the facts, it is very important to talk about our feelings. Having a support network of friends and family is imperative. These people are important not just for listening or giving advice but for providing support, both tangible and intangible. (In the same way, when things are going well for us, we need to lend a hand to others.) In my church, and sometimes at work, when someone is seriously ill, people take turns preparing meals and taking them to the family. Patients who are recovering from bypass surgery tell me gratefully of a neighbor who mowed their lawn without even being asked. Such acts of kindness have physical value because they provide needed help, but they also have psychological value because they tell the recipient that they are not alone but have the support of others in their suffering.

When someone has a serious illness, others are often afraid to ask about it. Not asking aggravates the isolation the sufferer feels. Asking about their illness shows that you care and are thinking about them. It also opens the door for them to talk with you about their feelings. When I know someone is going through a hard time, I want to know how they are dealing with it, both to support them and to learn lessons that they may be able to teach me.

For the person who is suffering, talking about the problem helps to release emotional tension that has built up inside. It can untangle thoughts and stop them from spinning around in circles. If you have to, tell a friend that you just need to talk for a while and that you don't want any advice, just a listening ear. You may just need a good cry by yourself, or with a close friend or family member.

Expressing and experiencing our emotions is not exclusively verbal. Much of the best art, music, poetry, and literature is born from the suffering of the artist. These works are most completely appreciated by those who have shared that suffering. The sufferer can find solace through this unspoken communion.

For many of us, our faith is central to dealing with suffering. The suffering is usually beyond our control, and the purpose for it is beyond our knowledge. Religious faith gazes into realms we cannot see with reason alone. Houses of worship provide an automatic support group. Clergy provide a resource for both encouragement and counseling. It has been said that "there are no atheists in foxholes." In other words, most people facing death end up believing in God in some way. If you are in a foxhole, it may be time to explore the questions that science and worldly wisdom can't answer.

A Christian Perspective

One of the reasons that the Bible remains on bestseller lists is that it addresses all types of human suffering. Even if you do not want to accept the Bible's viewpoint on religious matters, you will find within its pages examples of human suffering that can illuminate your own experience. It is partly for this reason that literary classics often contain allusions to biblical stories. If you don't know the Bible, ask someone who does if there are some stories or some passages in the Bible that relate to your situation.

If you are in a foxhole, or any other deep hole, looking for a way out, be careful not to reach for just any rope that someone throws down. Examine the claims of any belief system or religion to determine whether they are credible. As a Christian, I believe that there is overwhelming historical evidence for the accuracy of the claims that Jesus made about himself. I also believe that Christianity is unique among world religions. While other religions expect human beings to save themselves, in Christianity God reaches out to us to give us grace and forgiveness. If you are in this situation of searching for answers, I would recommend that you read *More Than a Carpenter* by Josh McDowell and *Mere Christianity* by C. S. Lewis.[1]

Another source of help in dealing with problems is books that have been written to help you, some of which have a Christian focus. One great Christian book that I found helpful when going through a difficult time is *When God Doesn't Make Sense* by James Dobson.[2] Resources like this can be very helpful in dealing with difficult experiences.

Other Tools to Deal with Stress

Some of us deal with stress using logic. Sitting down with a piece of paper and planning how to deal with upcoming issues brings a sense of control. This step is important for everyone at some point. It gives us a chance to reconsider our priorities in light of the new facts that have been thrust into our consciousness.

Some of us use physical exercise to relieve stress. If our health allows, regular exercise can help maintain physical and emotional strength for the ordeal.

If you have tried all of this and are still paralyzed, the next step may be professional help from a counselor, psychologist, or psychiatrist. These individuals are trained to help you gain a perspective on your circumstances and to teach you how to function. Sometimes your reaction to a problem is exaggerated because of an unresolved conflict elsewhere in your life, and counseling may help you to see that. Often we need help to understand ourselves and why we react the way we do. A patient of mine became preoccupied with his cardiac risk after he lost a sibling to a stroke. He recognized that his preoccupation was not rational, but at times it was overpowering. After a few meetings with a psychologist, he regained a proper perspective and had no further problems.

Remember Mr. Phillips, the man with high blood pressure? He had accessed all these forms of support, and he was still unable to function. His reaction was so far beyond the usual reaction that I suspected he had a chemical imbalance in his brain that was disabling. Antidepressant medication finally allowed him to get back to a normal life.

Modern antidepressants are not addicting. Typically, if someone who is not depressed takes an antidepressant,

A Christian Perspective

When I go through difficult times, my Christian faith provides the most important answers and gives me the encouragement I need. Let me explain.

First, it gives purpose where there seems to be no purpose. We are promised in Romans 8:28–29 that "God causes all things to work together for good to those who love God, to those who are called according to His purpose. For whom He foreknew, He also predestined to be conformed to the image of His Son." These verses do not say that God causes bad things to happen. Bad things can happen for many reasons, or for no reason we can see. But the scripture does say that *when* those bad things happen, God causes them to bring about good. How? By helping us to grow in character, so that we can be "conformed to the image of His Son." In other words, we become more like God's Son. When I respond correctly, bad experiences make me more compassionate, more sensitive to others, more able to cope with adversity. Bad experiences refocus my priorities and inspire me to help others.

Believing this promise is important to me. Even when I cannot *see* how

it has very little effect. If someone is depressed, however, antidepressants can result in dramatic improvement.

Depression distorts reality so that we do not see things as they really are. Ellen Vaughn, in her excellent book *Radical Gratitude*, describes the effect of antidepressants as similar to putting on glasses.[3] These medications are not happy pills; they simply allow a depressed person to see more clearly, instead of through the fogged glass of depressive illness.

anything good can come out of a particular experience, I trust that God will use it to accomplish his purposes for me.

The second way that my Christian faith helps me through bad experiences is much more concrete. Any emotion I feel has been expressed eloquently somewhere in the Bible. The book of Psalms in particular contains honest expressions of many emotions, some of which are quite different from what you might expect. For example, in a number of psalms the writer asks God to make his enemies suffer. It is true that in our conduct we are to turn the other cheek and that in our attitudes we are to love our enemies, but God still wants us to *express our emotions* and has given us the writers of the psalms as our examples. When I am going through a bad time, I try to find a psalm that expresses my strongest feelings. I memorize that psalm, or that part of a psalm, and quote it to God to express my feelings to him. This practice is more therapeutic than you can imagine until you have tried it. Often the verses around the emotional ones provide insight into the lessons I need to learn, but whether this is the case or not, I am able to express my emotions more completely than I could otherwise.

Kubler-Ross's Stages

Perhaps you have not suffered the anxiety that made Carrie Compton so resistant to medicine or the terror that paralyzed Michael Phillips, but you are still struggling with a boiling pot of different feelings. Understanding the normal range of emotions associated with illness can help us get through the experience.

When we face a new problem of these proportions, it is normal to pass through a series of emotions. In 1969,

Elisabeth Kübler-Ross defined five stages of dealing with difficult situations in her book *On Death and Dying*.[4] The stages she described were denial, anger, bargaining, depression, and acceptance. Of course, you might go through six stages instead, or you might experience only four and go through them over and over in different orders. All of us do not go through these five stages in the same order. The point is that experiencing a series of emotions is normal. Understanding our emotions can free us to see more clearly and to separate the facts from our emotional response.

Denial

Denial is the stage when I do not want to believe that I have a problem. "I don't really have high blood pressure. Can we check it again next month?" Sometimes, with medical problems that are not urgent, our doctors may choose to do confirmatory tests to help us face a diagnosis. Sometimes I may be right that I do not have a problem. However, if I do have a problem, sooner or later I have to face it.

When someone is in denial, they will have a lot of anxiety about subjecting their body to treatment. Their body, like Carrie's, screams, "Why are you doing this to me? I don't even have high blood pressure [or cancer, or heart disease, or whatever is being treated]!"

Denial often delays proper care, with disastrous consequences. If someone is having a heart attack and comes to the hospital within an hour of the onset of symptoms, doctors can often open the blocked artery so that there will be no significant damage to the heart. If someone comes in after twenty-four hours, the damage is often completed. The risk of death or disability is then profound.

You probably know of someone who told their family after supper that they "just didn't feel well" and went up to bed early. The next morning, the family found their lifeless body. Some people delay getting help until it is too late.

"I know I'm having chest pain, but it's probably not my heart."

But what if it is?

"The pain will probably go away in a little while. I'll be fine in the morning."

What if you're wrong?

"If I go to the emergency room and it's not my heart, I'll look foolish."

It's better to look foolish than to *be* foolish.

When we are young and healthy and exercising to try to get in shape, it is often good to ignore pain. As we get older, ignoring pain becomes a weakness rather than a strength. Pay attention to your body. If something does not seem right, it makes sense to check it out rather than to take a chance.

We can also be afflicted by the opposite of denial. Sometimes we have anxiety because we believe we have a diagnosis that the doctor assures us we do not have. ("I know this headache is from a tumor.") Often confirmatory tests in that context are helpful and worth their cost in the long run, because otherwise we would keep seeking medical attention because we are not convinced that we are well. You may remember Cindy in chapter 2, who was told by a dishonest doctor that she had a serious heart condition, or Father Corapi, who was told by two dishonest doctors that he needed bypass surgery. Father Corapi saw multiple doctors before he was sure that the first doctors were lying. Cindy needed a lot of reassurance from me that her heart was normal before she could accept it.

Anger

Anger means that we are angry that we have a health problem. That anger may be directed at the doctor, at God, at ourselves, or at whoever is in our path at the time. When I was an intern, my patients generally appreciated me. Once, however, after a patient was diagnosed with cancer by the oncologist who had seen her at our request, the family became belligerent toward me and the other residents involved in her care, getting angry and argumentative about small things that would not have bothered them before. At the same time, they were very warm toward the oncologist. I recognized that they were letting their anger out at me, even though I had done nothing wrong. Knowing that their long-term relationship with the oncologist was more important, I was happy to fill the role of lightning rod if it would help them to get along with the oncologist better.

Maybe your parent is treating you the same way when you help them get medical care or insist that they get treatment. If so, recognize that this is usually a stage that people pass through.

Bargaining

Bargaining is the stage when we are willing to accept our situation but want either to get out of it or to minimize its effects through certain conditions.

- "I know I will die from this cancer, but I just want to live long enough to attend my son's wedding."
- "If God will let me live, I promise to serve him the rest of my life."

Kübler-Ross pointed out that most of her patients, if they got their request, usually tried to add more conditions:

- "I have another son who isn't married yet!"
- "I know I said I would serve God, but I think I should do some other things first."

This certainly proves that having a terminal illness does not stop us from being human.

I often see bargaining when a patient draws a line in the sand and does not want to cross it:

- "I'll take the medicines I'm on now, but I don't want to take any more medicines."
- "I'll take these medicines, but I never want to have surgery."
- "I'll try to lose weight, but I'm not giving up my cigarettes or my ice cream."

Before you draw a line in the sand, make sure you know what is on both sides of the line. No one wants to take medicines, or have surgery, or give up ice cream. The reason doctors end up recommending such things is that the consequences of a health problem in a given individual would be worse than the consequences of the treatment.

Depression

In the *depression* stage, we recognize that the problem is indeed real and is not going away, and it crushes us. We may become paralyzed by fear or anxiety, as Carrie was. We may be tearful, as many people are at this stage. We regret the things we have not done or the things we have done. We do not know how to go on from here, and we feel we cannot make it. For most people, this is a transient phase. When we become stuck in this phase, we should pursue the help discussed earlier.

Acceptance

Acceptance is the stage when we come to terms with the diagnosis. We accept that it is true and reconcile ourselves to dealing with it as well as we can. This is the ultimate healthy response. If you start here and don't have to go through other emotions, you're unusual. If after you come to acceptance, you don't go back and experience other emotions at times anyway, you're even more unusual.

For Carrie, after analyzing the facts, it was reasonable to reach the stage of acceptance, since high blood pressure is not a terminal illness. Unfortunately, for some people, analyzing the facts is more frightening. Remember Julie, who had the heart attack in chapter 1? Her major heart attack left her with a severely weakened heart. Unfortunately, she has a substantial risk of death in the next year. When she analyzes the facts, she has great reason to fear, get angry, and bargain. For her, the focus has to be on the fact that there is hope that she will do well and that in case she does not do well, she must do all she can to live each day to the fullest. She must also decide what she believes about life and death and come to terms with her situation and her beliefs.

Hope

After discussing these five responses to bad news, Ross goes on to say that *hope* persists through all of the feelings. Hope for a last-minute cure, hope for relief of symptoms, hope that tomorrow will be a better day, hope that our life will have a positive impact. Hope does not mean that we are unrealistic. It means that we know that there are things beyond our knowledge. It means that we know that anything is possible. Hope helps us get through the most difficult situations, and it is to be encouraged and nurtured in the worst of times.

When I need to tell a patient about their poor prognosis, I always try to hold out hope.

"Because your heart condition is so serious, we know that you have a 50 percent chance of dying in the next two years. Of course, we are going to do everything we can to be sure that you are in the *other* 50 percent."

"Things don't look good at all for your father. It looks like he's dying. Of course, I hope I'm wrong and things turn around and get better, but you should definitely call anyone who would want to see him and let them know that he may die, maybe even before morning."

The central importance of hope was articulated seven hundred years ago. In Dante's classic work *The Divine Comedy*, the entrance to hell is inscribed with the words "Abandon hope all ye who enter here." To Dante, the essence of hell was not just the suffering but the complete loss of hope. There is no reason to take hope away from yourself or from your loved ones. We must refuse false hope to avoid deception. But we must cling to true hope of some type, even if we know that we are terminally ill.

Summary

In this chapter, we have considered the range of emotions that we experience when facing illness. I have discussed how to understand these emotions and how to deal with them. I have reviewed healthy and unhealthy responses. But let me say on a personal note that I am sorry that you or your loved one is facing a health problem. I wish that my words could take away the problem, or at least take away the pain. But I know that no book that I may write, no words I may pen, no thought I may convey, will restore what you have lost.

Hopefully, this chapter has helped you deal with emotional issues, but you probably also have practical, physical problems I have not yet addressed. I will discuss those in the next chapter.

Notes

1. Josh McDowell, *More Than a Carpenter* (Carol Stream, Ill.: Tyndale, 1977); C. S. Lewis, *Mere Christianity* (New York: Macmillan, 1971).

2. James Dobson, *When God Doesn't Make Sense* (Carol Stream, Ill.: Tyndale, 1993).

3. Ellen Vaughn, *Radical Gratitude* (Grand Rapids: Zondervan, 2005), 128.

4. Elisabeth Kübler-Ross, *On Death and Dying* (New York: Macmillan, 1969).

13

✚

Frequently Asked Questions

"Dr. Brown, we have covered a lot of ground. I still have some questions. You may have answered some of them, but I just need to get a lot of these principles together."

"Julie, sometimes the best way to put things together is to ask questions."

After reading the preceding twelve chapters, you have learned a lot about health care, but you may be trying to apply it to some aspects of your situation and having difficulty. Maybe you tried to do some of the things I suggested and they didn't work. Maybe I haven't given you enough information to help with your particular problem. Maybe you just skipped to this chapter for some quick answers. Whatever your situation, let's look at some difficult and frequent problems and discuss how to deal with them.

When the Doctor Tells You Something You Don't Want to Hear

When we hear bad news, all of us want to awaken and discover we were just dreaming.

"There must be some mistake!"

"There must be some other way to get better besides surgery!"

"The doctor must be wrong!"

Today, if we type a diagnosis into a search engine on the Internet, we get thousands of links to websites that promise an easy cure without surgery or "dangerous drugs"—and far fewer links to sites that offer accurate and helpful information. When I see these false claims, even when I know that medically they are false, I *wish* that they were true. I am sure that you have seen, as I have, individuals who have believed these messages and have suffered as a result.

We are particularly vulnerable when we are in the emotional stage of denial. Happy messages are seductive. *Do not let yourself be easy prey to quacks and charlatans.* As discussed in earlier chapters, if there is an easy way out, your doctor will probably know it. And as we have seen, even the rich, the smart, and the famous can be deceived.

Coretta Scott King, civil rights leader and widow of the great Martin Luther King Jr., died at a clinic in Mexico in January 2006. She had been battling ovarian cancer. About a week later, the Mexican government shut down the clinic, stating that the clinic was operating without government authorization. The clinic had been founded and directed by Kurt W. Donsbach, an unlicensed chiropractor who, according to Stephen Barrett, has a long history of illegally promoting ineffective treatments.[1] Each of us is vulnerable if we do not investigate the facts about those we go to for our health care.

If you have cancer, or heart disease, or even high blood pressure, and someone tells you that they can solve your problem with no risk, how likely is that to be true? If you doubt the diagnosis, get a second opinion. If you do not like the proposed treatment, ask the doctor about alternatives or get a second opinion about that issue as well. But do not rely on the Internet or advertisements in a magazine to obtain accurate personal health advice. And if a clinic staffed by U.S. citizens is located outside the United States, there is probably a reason other than the weather.

I've Tried Conventional Medicine, and I Am No Better.

There are some conditions for which conventional medicine is not very effective. Incurable cancers are one category. There is also a larger category, however, of conditions that are not life threatening but have a huge impact on quality of life. Low back pain, chronic fatigue syndrome, and fibromyalgia are all good examples. Autism is another powerful example, with parents who are desperate for anything that might help. Conventional therapies are of some benefit for these disorders, but most individuals are left with a lot of symptoms and a lessened quality of life. If you have one of these conditions, you may figure that you have nothing to lose by trying unconventional treatment. Unfortunately, that is not true.

Don't forget that every treatment that may be helpful also has the potential to be harmful, albeit typically in a small percentage of people. This risk is present even when doctors use approved drugs in unproven ways. With no evidence, for example, some practitioners have treated fibromyalgia and chronic fatigue syndrome with prolonged courses of antibiotics. This process kills the normal flora in the digestive tract and can thereby lead to life-threatening diarrhea and bleeding. Risks are also present with untested supplements, even though these risks are often undefined.

Pursuing such treatments is also a waste of your resources, spiritually, emotionally, and physically. It would be better to focus on treatments that have promise or proven effectiveness, even if they help you only a little. When these treatments are exhausted, why not enroll in experimental trials, where potential treatments are being rigorously tested? Even if this does not help you, it will help others. Further, institutional review boards oversee clinical trials. These boards ensure that the research is ethical, minimizing your risk of harm and maximizing your chances of benefit.

There is a wise saying in Proverbs 27:6: "Faithful are the wounds of a friend, but deceitful are the kisses of an enemy." Disappointing truth is better than false hope. It is better to know the truth that no one knows what to do for your condition, so that you can adjust to it, than to chase all over the world or all over the Internet to look for something that isn't there. Your example for others, including your children, is more important than you can imagine.

There is an observation among doctors that patients with cancer are among the nicest people we meet. Perhaps that is because they have looked at their own mortality and have a better perspective on what is important in life and what is unimportant. When faced with an illness we cannot overcome, we have an opportunity to realize what has been true all along: we have no real control over our lives. Sure, we can alter our *risks* by taking care of ourselves and seeking the best medical care. But in the end, sooner or later, we will age, we will become ill, and we will die. For some of us that time comes sooner, and for others it comes later. But eventually it comes for all of us. This realization should allow us to make the best of our situation and to focus on what is truly important in the context of our struggles. We may not live as long or as easily as we had hoped, but we can live *better* than we had hoped.

I've Been to Five Different Doctors, and No One Can Tell Me What's Wrong.

If you find yourself in this situation, there are several possibilities, and each needs to be carefully and honestly considered. The first possibility is that you have not found the right doctor. Certainly by this point you should have already seen someone who specializes in whatever the problem seems to be. These specialists, even if they do not know the answer, will be able to recommend other doctors in the same or different specialties for further evaluation. If they have not done so, speak to a nurse in the doctor's office and ask if there is anyone else you could see who might be able to shed more light on the problem. If your doctors have no recommendations, a major university with a medical school is usually a good place to find doctors familiar with the latest medical breakthroughs.

A second possibility is that you have a condition that is not yet recognized by medical science. This possibility is unlikely, but new diseases are described from time to time, so it is possible. Of course, this may not help you much, but at least it is an answer.

Some types of chronic pain fall into this category. Doctors can exclude dangerous causes quite well, but some people are left with the pain and no explanation. That is why there is a new specialty, pain medicine, to help people in that category. These doctors specialize in treating chronic pain, even when no specific reason can be identified by other doctors. Sometimes they know of newer explanations beyond the knowledge of other physicians. Other times they may not have an explanation, but they are able to help.

A third possibility is that there is a psychological aspect to your symptoms. Does that mean you're crazy? No, it does not. Depression and anxiety can manifest themselves in many physical ways. Even when they are not the primary cause of symptoms, they play a role in how we experience them.

Even if your doctors believe that there is a psychological component to your symptoms, they may not tell you. There are a number of reasons for this. For one thing, they do not want to offend you. They would prefer that someone else deliver the news, even if it is true. They want you to know that they took the possibility of a physical cause seriously and that they are not dismissing you as crazy. They also do not want to ascribe your symptoms to a psychological cause unless they are confident that all possible physical causes have been excluded. In addition, even if the psychological possibility is explored, they will need to investigate further if there is any worsening in symptoms. Sometimes a physical cause may not be evident on first examination, but when symptoms worsen, a physical cause becomes obvious.

When I was a child, I heard a story about a woman who went to her doctor with some health problems. The doctor told her that her symptoms were "all in her head." A few months later, her symptoms worsened, and a second doctor diagnosed a brain tumor.

This occurred before the days of CAT scanning, so diagnosis of brain tumors was more difficult then than now. When I became a doctor, I realized that diagnosing the brain tumor might well have been impossible when she went to the first doctor, but obvious by the time she saw the second. For that reason, when we have finished testing for a given symptom, I always tell the patient, "We have not found a dangerous cause at this point, but if your symptoms worsen or change somehow, you need to let us know so that we can reassess your problem."

If you have had a thorough evaluation with no explanation for your symptoms, ask the doctor if there might be a psychological component to your symptoms. You should ask the same question of yourself and consider whether you have been depressed or anxious about your problems. With health problems, an emotional response is normal, and sometimes it is hard to distinguish cause from effect. Sometimes it is best to see a psychiatrist to determine whether there is a psychological component. Sometimes it is appropriate to try taking an antidepressant for a month or so to see if it helps.

If you agree that there may be a psychological component to your symptoms, you may think, "I should be able to work through this." If you were home having a heart

A Christian Perspective

As a Christian, I would add the possibility that a health problem, or the symptoms associated with it, may have a *spiritual* cause. For example, guilt and bitterness can cause a lot of physical problems, and they can worsen symptoms of medical diseases. While psychological problems can come from physical causes, such as chemical imbalances in the brain, they can also arise from unresolved conflicts in our relationships with ourselves, with others, and with God. The solution to these conflicts is spiritual, such as giving or receiving forgiveness. Counseling can help uncover these conflicts and help you find solutions.

attack, you would not try to work through it on your own. In the same way, if you are truly depressed, you will not be able to work through that chemical imbalance on your own any more than you can work through the heart attack. Do not be afraid of taking medication to correct what may be simply a different kind of physical problem, one that manifests itself in your mood.

Something that should be of comfort: if you have had a thorough evaluation with no answers, you can be reassured first that you probably do not have a life-threatening problem. Modern medicine is very good at diagnosing cancers, blocked arteries, and organ failure. Many problems that are not life threatening are harder to diagnose and are not as well understood.

I Just Can't Take Medicines. They All Give Me Side Effects.

I sure hope that you're wrong, because if you aren't, you won't live as long as you could have. Do you really think that you're so beyond the ordinary that you can't take any of the medicines that make other people live longer? All of us have the potential to have side effects with any medicine. Some people have true allergic reactions, such as itching and rashes, to multiple medications. But all of our bodies work in similar ways. That is why medications can help so many different people. Remember the story of Carrie Compton in chapter 12 and how she misinterpreted her symptoms as being due to her medications.

Don't forget the "nocebo" effect, where someone believes that the medication caused a problem for them when in reality the problem has nothing to do with the medication. When you have a problem that you think might be caused by a medication, ask your doctor whether the problem might be related to the medicine. Your doctor may tell you that your problem is probably related to the medicine. Alternatively, your doctor may tell you that he is not sure, and he may have you stop the medication to see if the problem goes away; then he may have you try starting the medication again to see if the problem comes back. Your doctor may also tell you that it is very unlikely that your problem is related to the medication. In this case, the next step is to look for other causes of your problem.

One patient told me that she was allergic to "all pain medications." I warned her that even if I believed that about myself, I certainly wouldn't tell anybody. If I had terrible pain one day, I would certainly want doctors to try to give me relief. We should have the same attitude about life-saving medications and be willing to try them when they may help us.

Why Not Do What the Conventional Doctor Tells Me Plus Use Alternative Medicine?

There is nothing wrong with this approach as long as you do it under the supervision of your physician and as long as you understand that there are risks involved in the alternative treatments. As discussed in earlier chapters, many times the specific risks of alternative treatments are not known, and often the potential interactions between "supplements" and conventional medications have not been studied. So even if your doctor consents, you are probably taking risks that your doctor cannot know or tell you about.

Still, your doctor may be able to tell you some of the risks and, in some cases, even some of the potential benefits of the alternative treatment. Unfortunately, the *established* benefits are usually much less than what the sellers of these products try to suggest.

I Can't Find a Good Doctor
like the Ones You've Described.

There are not many evil doctors, but there are an awful lot of mediocre doctors. As our society has become more selfish and more "me oriented," fewer and fewer people have the commitment to service that is necessary to provide the best medical care. Unless something dramatic changes in our society, this problem will only get worse. In addition, no one is perfect. You will not find a perfect doctor, anymore than you will find a perfect anything else.

You should certainly look as widely as you can to find the best doctor that you can. That may require looking in nearby towns or going a significant distance to see a specialist if you have a serious health problem. You may have to settle for less than your ideal. Once you have found the best doctor you can, use the principles in chapter 4 to build a strong relationship with that person and his or her staff. If you have questions about health issues as the years go by, you will have a strong enough relationship to ask more questions or to request referrals for additional input or second opinions on your care.

I Am Actually Very Happy with My Health Care,
but My Family and Friends Want Me to Pursue
Alternative Treatments.

I hear about this problem quite often in my practice. It is nice to have people who love us and want the best for us. Because they love us, they want a risk-free solution for our health problems. Unfortunately, risk-free solutions do not exist. If you can get these individuals to read this book, it will help them understand health care in a way they do not now.

If you have not had this problem, you may think you can just tell people it's none of their business. Perhaps sometimes that's appropriate. But in general, people suggest alternative treatments with the best of intentions. If the treatments they suggest are not of value, you may be able to refer them to a website like www.quackwatch.com to show them the facts. Sometimes they may be suggesting a different conventional treatment or an alternative treatment that you cannot find on Quackwatch. If so, discuss their suggestion with your doctor, and bring your loved one along if that is appropriate. Then the issues can be aired openly and fully with expert, individualized advice. It may even turn out that they have a good idea.

After this discussion, if you decide not to pursue the course of action they recommend, you can let them know that you do not want to discuss it further.

What Do I Do When I Can't Afford My Medicine or My Doctor's Visits, or I Can't Afford a Recommended Treatment?

Discuss this with your doctor. You are not the only one in this situation, and I can guarantee your doctor has faced this problem before.

When the issue is medications, your doctor can often provide samples. There are pharmaceutical company prescription-assistance programs that may be able to help. Most communities also have programs to help with medications. It is often possible to use a less expensive medication, and this may be the simplest solution.

If the problem is the ability to pay your doctor, I have never heard of a doctor's office that does not allow people to set up a payment plan, often without charging interest.

I Don't Want to Have to Take Pills for the Rest of My Life.

Mrs. Abbott was eighty-two years old when she came to see me because of difficulty with controlling high blood pressure. Her hair was short and gray. She needed a cane to get around but had still managed to be fairly independent. We talked about her numerous children, grandchildren, great-grandchildren, and the one great-great-grandchild who was anticipated. We discussed the nature of high blood pressure and how we would be treating it. I gave her some samples of a new medicine to take. Then she stopped me.

"Dr. Brown, I don't understand. I've never had to take medication before."

A few years ago, I looked into the mirror and discovered that I no longer had just the odd gray hair. It is still not all gray, or even mostly gray, but there is enough gray that no one thinks I'm thirty. My metabolism is also a lot slower than it used to be. If I eat the same quantities of food that I ate when I was in medical school, I will gain weight faster than those guys on television at the hot-dog-eating contests.

When a teenager looks at someone their parents' age, they assume that person is fundamentally different from themselves. When a parent who is thirty-five looks at their parent who is sixty, they think that their parent is fundamentally different from themselves. One of the great revelations we get as we age is that even though we grow older on the outside, we don't grow older on the inside. The ninety-year-old grandmother, whose skin is wrinkled and leathery, whose eyes are clouded by macular degeneration and cataracts, who has to get her granddaughter to help pluck away her facial hair, who leaves her teeth in a jar at night, who has to take nitroglycerin tablets for chest pain, is no different on the inside from the way she was the evening her future husband pinned on her corsage for the prom.

"What a beautiful concept," you think. Well, it is a beautiful concept when you apply it to other people. But it is harder to swallow when applied to ourselves. Even though I don't think of myself differently, that gray hair growing out of my head is still my own, though it used to be dark brown. When I trip and fall, I know I will be sorer for a longer period of time than I would have been (gasp) twenty years ago. And in all probability, one day I, like you, will be sitting in a doctor's office being told that I have high blood pressure, or cancer, or heart disease.

Sooner or later, we all develop health problems. When that happens, instead of resisting the pills or the surgery that we need, we should be grateful that these treatments are available. As noted earlier, life expectancy increased by thirty years during the twentieth century. Without these medicines and surgeries, our lives would be shorter and our quality of life would be worse.

Sure, it is easier to accept that thought intellectually than it is to accept it emotionally. And I don't think getting a sports car will help in the long run, even though it might make you feel better in the short run.

I do believe that these reminders of our mortality should motivate us to do the important things. They have certainly motivated me to write this book. They also motivate me to spend time with my family. They encourage me to treat others well and to make each day count.

Of course you don't want to take pills for the rest of your life. No one does. But if the alternative is an increased risk of stroke, or death from cancer or another health problem, then taking the pills is the best option.

Note

1. Stephen Barrett, "Donsbach's Clinic Closed; Victim Files Suit," *Consumer Health Digest* 6 (2006): 1. This is an e-mail newsletter, available for viewing at www.ncahf.org/digest06/06-06.html (accessed July 3, 2006). There are additional details about Donsbach's history in Stephen Barrett, "The Shady Activities of Kurt Donsbach," 2006, www.quackwatch.org/01QuackeryRelatedTopics/donsbach.html (accessed July 3, 2006).

14

✛

How Can I Live a Healthy Life?

"Dr. Brown, I think I've asked all of my questions about illness. But I also want to know how to stay healthy and what attitudes I should have about my health."

"Julie, there are a lot of principles that are simple but too often ignored. We need to follow those principles, and we need to keep health issues in proper perspective. If we do, we will make our journey through health care, and our journey through life, a lot more pleasant."

I hope that by now I have addressed the immediate health concerns that made you buy this book. But how can we maintain our health? And how do we put our health in perspective relative to other issues in our lives? In this chapter, I will start by discussing some simple things that all of us can and should do but too often don't do. Then

I will discuss some ideas that I think will help you live a more complete life in the context of illness.

Avoid Unhealthy Habits

Maintain Your Ideal Body Weight

Emma was sixty-five years old when I met her. At that point she was a little over five feet tall, if you could call it "tall" when she had to be measured lying in bed. She was no longer able to stand and had terrible pain when she even tried to sit up. She weighed over 300 pounds.

Ten years before, she weighed 234 pounds. She had injured her knee in a fall, and x-rays showed arthritis in her knees, hips, and spine. Her doctor warned her that if she did not lose weight, she would end up in a wheelchair. Little did her doctor know that this warning was overly optimistic. She lost about ten pounds with Weight Watchers, then got off the program. At the time she was able to do some walking, and this helped her maintain her weight. Then, about five years ago, she fell and broke her hip. After that she was able to walk only with a walker. Even though her activity decreased, she was just as hungry, and her food intake did not change.

As she continued to gain weight, it became harder to use her walker. Eventually, she got around exclusively in a wheelchair. Finally, it was too hard to get into her wheelchair. Now she was in bed all the time. She had a catheter in her bladder to drain the urine. She wore diapers in case an aide did not get to her in time with the bedpan. In spite of the best efforts of her caregivers in the nursing home, she smelled the way you would expect her to, from a mixture of her own waste and the sweat that dried under her many folds of skin.

Her daughter, Amanda, still brought the grandchildren to visit, but they never stayed with her for more than a few minutes. Even though she longed to see them more, she couldn't blame them. Amanda herself did not visit as much as she had in the past. She was overweight as well. Emma knew that seeing her scared her daughter. She hoped that it scared her enough to make her lose weight now, while it was easier.

Emma is an extreme example of one of the most common health problems in our society: obesity. It causes damage to the liver, the bones, and the joints. Because it raises blood pressure, blood sugar, and cholesterol, and because it promotes inactivity, it leads to heart disease, stroke, and diseases in blood vessels all over the body.

A significant proportion of people around the world today live in hunger, with too little food to eat. The United States, on the other hand, has so much excess food that we have to tell people to eat less. Restaurants are criticized for giving their customers too much food for the money.

You may think that Emma is an extreme case, and indeed she is. But the next time you look at someone who is more overweight than you are and wonder how they got that way, remember that the answer to that question is always "One bite at a time." Most people don't end up as big as Emma, but most people end up a lot bigger than they ever thought they would.

Even being slightly overweight has adverse health consequences. Most of my patients are overweight. Usually their health problems are not caused by obesity, but obesity makes them worse. Most of my patients would need less medicine for their blood pressure and cholesterol, and some of them could get off medication altogether, if they would lose weight.

How do we gain or lose weight? There is no magic to it. Weight is just like money. If you spend more money than you take in, your bank account will shrink. If you save more than you spend, your bank account will grow larger. If you eat more calories than you burn, you gain weight. If you burn more calories than you eat, you lose weight. With both money and weight, small changes maintained over a long period of time pay off in a bigger way than quick changes over a short period of time. The twenty-year-old who saves three dollars a week comes out way ahead of the sixty-year-old who suddenly starts trying to save thousands of dollars a month for retirement.

Our bodies try very hard to maintain the weight that we have. If you decided to eat nothing but carrots but ate as many as you wanted, you would tend to take in enough carrots to maintain your weight. Therefore, portion control is the only way to lose weight and maintain the loss. By far, the most successful program that works long term is Weight Watchers. It is a program that even teaches you what to do when you go out to eat. It also teaches you to control your portion sizes. The emphasis is on lifelong weight control. Unfortunately, the sad truth is that if you are overweight, you need to continue to follow a weight-loss program for the rest of your life or you will tend to regain the weight.

There are plenty of fad diets and new books out there with systems that may help you lose weight in the short run. What you really need is a program that you can and will follow long term. Then, you have to make up your mind to follow it.

As we get older, our metabolism gets slower, and it becomes harder to lose pounds. We have to take in fewer and fewer calories just to maintain our weight without gaining. If you wait until you are immobile, it will be even harder, because then you cannot increase the number of calories that you burn.

That is the other side of the equation. Increasing your burning of calories through exercise helps you lose weight.

However, as discussed above, your body will tend to take in enough calories to maintain your weight. So if you do not limit your calorie intake, exercise alone will not lead to much weight loss.

For Emma, it is too late to salvage mobility. She has destroyed her ability to get around. She has destroyed her chances to really know and play with her grandchildren. She has shortened her life and has left her daughter with sad memories of her fixed to her bed. She has spent her life savings and cost society thousands of dollars paying for caregivers to lift and turn her massive body.

Stop Smoking

Alice Moseley was only forty-five years old when she came in with a massive heart attack. She looked at least fifteen years older, the result of smoking three packs of cigarettes a day for many years. She had blockages in all three of the arteries to her heart and was sent to emergency bypass surgery. She was in shock for several days afterward, and it looked like she would die. When she came out of shock, she was still dependent on the breathing machine. This was partly due to her emphysema, which she did not know she had before, and partly due to a condition called adult respiratory distress syndrome (ARDS). This condition can develop in people who go into shock. It makes the lungs stiff, so that it takes more force to inflate them. People with ARDS are often dependent on a breathing machine for weeks or even months.

Every day, I would discuss Mrs. Moseley's critical illness with her family. She was on the ventilator for weeks. When it looked as if she would finally be able to get off the ventilator, she developed pneumonia and was on the ventilator for another month. Eventually, we got her off the ventilator, and after another two months of care in the hospital and at an inpatient rehabilitation unit with intensive physical therapy, she came to see me in the office.

"Are you staying off the cigarettes?"

"Oh, you don't have to worry about that, Dr. Brown. After what I've been through, I will never light up again."

Two months later, she was back in the office, and I smelled cigarette smoke. She had also stopped taking her cholesterol medicine.

"Mrs. Moseley, what happened? Two months ago, you swore you'd never touch cigarettes again."

"I really like smoking, Dr. Brown."

"This may sound unkind, but how do you feel about breathing? I spent months nursing you back from the edge

A Christian Perspective

The view of God as a cosmic concierge who lets you pick and choose what you want, and does whatever you ask, is not consistent with God's character. You cannot pick the bits you want and leave the rest. If you are going to trust God with your health, you need to follow his direction in all areas. Of course you will fail at times. We are all imperfect. But to expect him to let you dictate the terms of your physical redemption is arrogant and sinful. If you want to be a good example to your doctors and the others around you, trust him to help you overcome your self-destructive habits and develop habits that will have a positive impact on your health.

Alice may be able to fool herself about this, but she will not fool her doctor. Christians who refuse sound medical advice and continue to engage in self-destructive habits do great damage to God's reputation.

of death, and your poor sons spent months watching you hooked up to a machine. Sooner or later, your smoking will put you back on that ventilator."

"I know, Dr. Brown, but it's just so hard to stop."

"By the way, why aren't you taking your cholesterol medicine?"

"Dr. Brown, I'm going to trust God to lower my cholesterol without medication."

"Why don't you trust him to help you stop smoking?"

"I don't know, Dr. Brown." She laughed. "I guess I should."

"Don't you think that God has provided cholesterol medications to help you get your cholesterol lower?"

"Maybe he has. But I don't like medicines."

"So let me get this straight. You want to trust God to allow you not to take pills, which you don't want to take anyway. But you don't want to trust him to help you get off the cigarettes because you enjoy smoking."

"I guess you're right, Dr. Brown. It doesn't make much sense, does it?"

Tobacco is one of the most damaging products to health that is available. If someone has a heart attack and stops smoking, they cut their risk of death in the next year *in half* compared with what it would be if they continued to smoke. And that is only the first year.

Smoking causes cancer, emphysema, heart disease, and stroke. It makes you smell bad, too. Smokeless tobacco causes cancer, especially of the tongue and lips. You may have seen one of those billboards that show someone with half of their face removed due to smokeless tobacco. Smokeless tobacco makes arteries squeeze down and in this way raises blood pressure.

Quitting is difficult. There are two aspects to the addiction to tobacco. The first is the physical addiction. If you can stay off cigarettes for three days, you are pretty much over the physical part. For people who cannot get through those three days, nicotine replacement therapies, such as the gums and patches, allow you to spread those three days out over several weeks or several months. If you're able to stay off for three days but then start back later, your problem is the psychological addiction. For most smokers, the psychological addiction is stronger than the physical addiction. There are a number of resources available from the American Cancer Society to help you fight the psychological addiction. There are also medications that can help considerably with the psychological addiction. You should discuss these options with your doctor.

Whatever you do, do it now. Our lungs are like many other organs in the body. You can lose 80 percent of your kidney function or 80 percent of your liver function, and never know the difference. But when you get down to that last 20 percent, every little bit makes a big difference. All of us lose lung function as part of the aging process. When you stop smoking, you stop the ongoing damage from the cigarettes, but you do not stop the loss of lung function that is part of the normal aging process. I have seen many patients suffer and die from emphysema even though they stopped smoking thirty years before, when they had no symptoms of lung disease. Unfortunately, when they quit smoking, they were already down to maybe 30 or 40 percent. Finally, through aging, they got down to that last 20 percent. Because they have reached this critical threshold, they feel like they have suddenly fallen off a cliff as they become out of breath at lower and lower levels of activity. Had they not quit smoking, they would have been in trouble a lot sooner, so they are still better off than they would have been. But nothing can bring back the lung tissue that they destroyed.

The bottom line: you can't stop smoking too soon, but you can certainly stop smoking too late.

Don't Drink Too Much

Some medical studies have found a lower risk of health problems in those who consume small amounts of alcohol. However, there are many confounding variables in these studies, so that consensus panels have *not* recommended that people drink alcohol for their health. If you choose to drink alcohol, there is a strong consensus that no woman should drink more than one to two drinks at a time and no man should drink more than one to three drinks at a time. Larger amounts damage the liver, the heart, and the brain. One drink would be defined as 1.25 ounces of liquor (not one tumbler full), one glass of wine, or 12 ounces of beer.

Alcohol impairs our ability to drive even at levels far less than the levels defined in "driving while intoxicated" statutes. Driving with alcohol in your system can cause devastating damage and destruction physically and emotionally, both to you and to others.

Don't Abuse Drugs

The variety of different drugs that are abused and their potential harm are well beyond the scope of this book. A simple summary is that if you are abusing drugs, legal or illegal, you need to stop if you want to protect your health.

Build Good Habits

Avoiding bad habits is the first step, but building good habits is almost as important. Good habits help to maintain health and provide an early-warning system to detect new problems early.

Pay Attention to Your Body

When a soldier is twenty years old and running down a battlefield, it is good for him to ignore pain, even if a bullet hits him. If he stops and stands still, he will be worse off than if he continues running until he gets to a safe place. On the other hand, when he is sixty and develops chest pain, ignoring it is no longer such a good idea, since his symptoms may be due to a serious heart problem.

As we age, it is important to notice changes in our body and to get them checked out. Breast self-examination is important for early detection of breast cancer. Testicular examination is important even in that twenty-year-old soldier to detect testicular cancer early. Symptoms that are new, including new moles, new bleeding problems, new shortness of breath, new chest discomfort—anything that is not explained completely by a brief viral illness—warrant a trip to see the doctor. As the saying goes, it's better to be safe than sorry. Vigilance is one of your best defenses against a new health problem.

Get Regular Exercise

If your doctor agrees that it is safe for you, you should be building a regular exercise program. The goal for heart health is to spend at least thirty minutes at least three times a week exercising hard enough to be short of breath. By that I mean exercising hard enough that it is hard to carry on a conversation.

As we age, we have less and less ability to get around and less and less stamina. The only thing that prevents this age-related decline is regular exercise, and the more vigorous, the better.

Most people who exercise get a warning before they have a heart attack. As blockages worsen, people typically develop symptoms that come on with exertion and go away with rest. Seeking medical attention when you notice this pattern can often prevent a heart attack, for the doctor can treat a blockage before the artery is totally blocked.

Decreasing exercise tolerance can be a sign of anemia, a lung problem, or even abnormal thyroid function. If you are not exercising and wait until you get symptoms at rest, the problem will be much more advanced and is more likely to be fatal or incurable.

Unless there is a medical problem that makes it dangerous, it is important to exercise even when it is difficult. Fatigue is one of the most common problems people report. Fatigue can be caused by many different problems, including cancer, so you need to discuss it with your doctor. However, in most people we do not find a dangerous cause. Exercise will help these people more than anything else.

"But I can't exercise. I'm too tired."

This decision leads to a downward spiral. Because of inactivity, exercise tolerance worsens, and we are more easily fatigued. It is important to turn the spiral around.

"Even though I'm too tired, I'm going to make myself exercise. If I can walk only one block, I'll try to do that twice a day. Maybe next week I can make it two blocks."

That kind of attitude will make you stronger and give you more energy. One of my patients told me that the hardest part of exercising was opening his front door. Once we get started and make it a priority, exercise helps us to stay healthy.

Weigh Yourself Every Day

We all tend to gain weight as we get older. If you discover that you have gained two or three pounds, it is not so hard to lose it. But if you gain ten or fifteen pounds, you have a much more difficult task. Weighing yourself daily allows you to know where you stand and to do something about it before you end up like Emma.

Follow Consensus Recommendations for Cancer Screening

See your primary care physician regularly and ask what you should be doing to prevent problems and detect them early. Professional medical societies have developed guidelines about what tests should be done at various ages. Your doctor should be familiar with these guidelines. It is also important to look at these consensus guidelines yourself.

For early detection of cancer, the American Cancer Society's guidelines tend to be more aggressive in terms of recommending screening tests than most. Their guidelines, like those of most such organizations, can be viewed on the Internet.[1] You probably know that breast examinations and mammography are important in the early detection of breast cancer. Hopefully, you also know that colonoscopy is important to detect colon cancer early. At present, it is recommended that all of us have our first colonoscopy at age fifty, or earlier if we have a family history of colon cancer or precancerous colon polyps. Unfortunately, this test is expensive and may not be covered by your insurance policy. However, it is very effective in preventing death from colon cancer. Pap smears for women and regular prostate examinations and blood tests for men are also important. Fortunately, these simpler tests are usually covered by insurance.

Your doctor can discuss with you how often your blood pressure and cholesterol levels should be checked and whether other tests are important for you. Regular ex-

A Christian Perspective

There are a lot of people out there who try to claim a biblical mandate for their own brand of health care, whether it is a diet or a supplement. Many of these claims are at best unorthodox, and at worst they are deliberate scams. But there are some principles in the Bible that are straightforward in their application and relate directly to our physical health.

Honor Your Parents

One of the Ten Commandments, recorded in Deuteronomy 5:16, tells us, "Honor your father and your mother, as the LORD your God has commanded you, that your days may be prolonged, and that it may go well with you on the land which the LORD your God gives you."

Did you catch that promise? This verse tells us that if we honor our father and mother, we will enjoy a long life. This teaching is like many principles in the Bible. It is not a *guarantee* that we will live to be ninety no matter how much we smoke. It is not a *guarantee* against automobile accidents or early serious illnesses. It does mean that if we honor our parents, we will live longer than we would if we did not honor them. Perhaps this is because we avoid unresolved conflicts that would otherwise dog us the rest of our days and lead to health problems. Perhaps it is because listening to our parents' practical advice protects us from harm we would otherwise face. Whatever the reason, I am happy to accept the promise as a matter of faith.

Keep a Clear Conscience

Psalm 32 contains observations about the physical effects of guilt.

> How blessed is he whose transgression is
>> forgiven,
> Whose sin is covered!
> How blessed is the man to whom the Lord does
>> not impute iniquity,
> And in whose spirit there is no deceit!
> When I kept silent about my sin, my body
>> wasted away
> Through my groaning all the day long.
> For day and night Your hand was heavy upon
>> me;
> My vitality was drained away as with the fever
>> heat of summer.
> I acknowledged my sin to You,
> And my iniquity I did not hide;
> I said, "I will confess my transgressions to the
>> Lord,"
> And You forgave the guilt of my sin. (vv. 1–4)

A guilty conscience makes our body waste away. It drains away our vitality. I once heard a preacher point out that the reason most people feel guilty is that they are guilty. If I have a guilty conscience, I need to seek forgiveness from God and from the person I have offended. It is very difficult to humble myself and ask forgiveness. However, the only thing harder in the long run than seeking forgiveness is not seeking forgiveness.

Be Merciful

We are warned in Proverbs 11:17 that "the merciful man does himself good, but the cruel man does himself harm."

The Bible teaches that if we are cruel to others, we are actually hurting ourselves. On the other hand, have you ever chosen to ignore it when someone wrongs you, deliberately extending unrequested forgiveness? That is mercy, and the Bible says that it is good for you.

What about doing something unexpectedly nice to someone for no reason at all? There is a special sense of freedom and joy in these unselfish acts. In the secular world, there has been a lot of talk about doing "random acts of kindness." If there were more of these, the world would certainly be a better place. According to this verse, the world would also be a *healthier* place. Just try it. Not only will you enjoy it, but the memory of the act will stay with you for years.

There are spiritual rewards also, as Matthew 5:7 promises: "Blessed are the merciful, for they shall receive mercy." I don't know about you, but when I stand before God, I want all the mercy I can get.

Be Righteous

Psalm 31:10 describes the results of living an unrighteous life:

> For my life is spent with sorrow
>
> And my years with sighing;
>
> My strength has failed because of my iniquity,
>
> And my body has wasted away.

Unrighteousness saps our strength. This is not a hard and fast rule but a general principle. There are plenty of evil people who live to a ripe old age and die comfortably in their beds, and plenty of good people who die young. However, the last two verses of this psalm promise:

> Oh, love the LORD, all you His godly ones!
>
> For the LORD preserves the faithful, and fully
>
> > recompenses the proud doer.
>
> Be strong and let your heart take courage,
>
> All you who hope in the LORD. (vv. 23–24)

Even if we do not see the positive results in this life, we will see them in the next.

aminations of your skin are also important to try to detect skin cancers early.

As discussed in earlier chapters, not every screening test is a good idea. When your doctor recommends a screening test, you should still ask about the data that support its use. Be at least a little suspicious if the cost is not covered by insurance, unless you are on Medicare, which severely limits the use of screening tests.

Eat a Healthy Diet

While there is a lot of uncertainty about whether various vitamins or supplements decrease our risk of problems, there is little controversy about eating a healthy diet. Even if it does not do as much good as we might hope, it is unlikely to do us any harm. A good diet is low in fat, especially saturated fat, and high in fiber. In short, eat lots of fruits and vegetables and not so much meat, cheese, nuts, and processed foods. Fish, especially darker-meat fishes like salmon and tuna, seems to be of particular benefit with respect to cardiac health. As discussed earlier, the amount of food we eat needs to be adjusted to achieve and maintain as close to our ideal body weight as possible.

Don't Expect Something for Nothing

When you hear about a new treatment or screening test that sounds too good to be true, be skeptical about it, and discuss it at length with your doctor. Do not be gullible about your health, any more than you would be gullible about your finances.

Learning from Illness

Experiences are unsettling when they upset our view of the world. For the most part, being unsettled means that we have learned that something we had assumed is not true. Let's look at the ways illness shatters our illusions.

This Body of Mine Will Not Last Forever.

Greg had looked forward to this day for the past thirty years. He had finally put in enough time at the factory to retire. This afternoon he would go to his retirement party. Tomorrow he and his wife would get into their truck and tow their camper to their favorite state park to begin his retirement travels. He had already planned the first six months. He had plans for fishing, camping, and visiting grandchildren from now until September. He figured that he and Rebecca would spend their winters in their house here. He had sketched out plans for a new kitchen he would build for her. He had also talked with Meals on Wheels about volunteering two days a week during the fall and winter.

As he worked on the assembly line, he began to feel a strange feeling in his chest. He had never felt anything quite like this before. Could it be his heart? He did not think so. He was only fifty-five. After half an hour, he had a break. In conversation with some of his buddies, he mentioned the strange sensation to them. They tried to get him to go to the hospital, but he didn't think it was necessary. Maybe it would go away if he waited.

He kept working, but it only got worse. Finally, at his next break, he let his friends call an ambulance, and they called his wife to let her know he was going to the hospital. His EKG in the emergency room showed that he was having a heart attack. He was taken to the heart catheterization laboratory with a plan for angioplasty. Just as he was being moved from the stretcher onto the x-ray table, his heart stopped. The doctors worked on him for an hour but never got his heart restarted.

As a doctor, I have an advantage over most people. Every time I see someone like Greg, I am reminded of my own mortality. I have no guarantee of tomorrow. That realization should affect the choices I make and the way I deal with others.

When we are young and healthy, the concept of death and decay seems like a nightmare in a mythical and far distant future. If you do not see people like Greg every day as I do, illness should remind you that death and decay will happen to you, too. When our body does not do what it should do, it shakes our world. When we hurt and have an unnatural awareness of our bodily functions, it should continually remind us of our mortal state.

I Do Not Have Control over My Body.

A man with arthritic hands said to me, "One day I looked down and realized that I no longer had my own hands, but my father's hands."

Aging works that way, and so does illness. Our blood pressure and cholesterol both rise with age. Cancers grow even though we did not plant them or give them our permission. Despite our best efforts, a clot forms in one of the arteries to our brain, and we suffer a stroke.

We certainly have some control over our health, and this book aims to help you maintain that control and minimize health problems. I can exercise and make my muscles stronger. I can eat badly and make my body fatter. But there are many things going on that are well beyond anything I can change. My hair turns gray. Arteries get blocked despite the best preventive care. Cancers grow.

Illness reminds us of this reality. Perhaps you have always tried to take good care of yourself, getting regular checkups and eating a healthy diet. Then one day, you discover that you have cancer that has already spread all over your body. You realize that despite your best efforts, an uninvited cancer has been growing inside you for a long time. Your body is no longer under your control.

In reality, your body has never been under your control. The rest of our life is not under our control either. I have a great idea to make money, and someone else markets it first. I lock my car and park next to the police station, but someone steals my radio anyway.

The idea that we control our life is an illusion. The sooner we realize that, the sooner we can deal with it.

A Christian Perspective

If you are a Christian, you should already know that God will use your illness for good, to make you more like Christ, as promised in Romans 8:28–29. You already know that you do not control your body. The Bible tells us explicitly, for example, that we cannot make ourselves taller by worrying (Matt. 6:27). It tells us that we cannot make even one hair white or black (Matt. 5:36). As a Christian, you also know that your mortal body will die. But knowing these things *in theory* is different from accepting them when you are the one who is facing death or illness. Faith means choosing to believe these truths in the midst of your suffering.

I Need to Decide What I Believe and Why.

Illness makes us face the central questions of human existence. What is the nature of God? What is the nature of humanity? Why am I here? Does life have a purpose?

I took a college English class in which we reviewed the work of a modern poet who addressed these questions. The professor was nearing retirement age. He remarked that he could understand if college students our age had not decided what we believed about these questions, but he thought it was foolish if someone his age had not decided what he believed.

In reality, even a college student can face death. We all need to decide what we believe about these questions. If you are facing death, disability, or serious illness, you know that this issue is important. If your illness is minor, you have still been reminded that we have little control over our lives, and that therefore we need to be ready to face death and to live wisely to make the most of whatever time we have. Be thankful for the illness that encourages you to answer life's important questions. The sooner you answer them and the more fully you face them, the better you will live your life.

If you have not decided what you believe, I would urge you to consider Christianity. Read *Mere Christianity* by C. S. Lewis,[2] or read the Bible itself, starting with the Gospel of John.

The "Me Generation"

When considering the meaning of life, the present generation focuses on self. This generation as a whole believes that life is all about *me*. My purpose on earth is to find happiness. It does not really matter whether that means divorcing my spouse and leaving my children behind. It does not really matter that I do not take responsibility for my parents. If I am in a situation that makes me unhappy, this philosophy would say, then I should get out.

This self-centered viewpoint makes my health one of my highest priorities. My goal is to avoid death and suffering for as long as possible. If you tell me that I will die and leave my pleasures behind no matter what I do, that is the ultimate bad news. If you tell me that I have to accept an imperfect body, with limitations in what I feel and what I can do, that is almost as bad. I want to stay young and fit forever. Because it is such a high priority, I will expend whatever resources I have to find the fountain of youth. I will read about the newest findings and travel the world to find the best treatments.

What Matters Most

Even though superficially our society has accepted this philosophy, underneath it still values self-sacrifice. Placing the welfare of others above ourselves is seen as heroic in our literature and in our films. Obi-Wan Kenobi in the Star Wars films and Neo in *The Matrix* are two examples from science fiction. In *Saving Private Ryan*, the squad of soldiers who rescue Private Ryan serve as a metaphor for all the soldiers in U.S. history who have given their lives to allow us to live in freedom.

Sometimes, the reasons for self-sacrifice are utilitarian. Charles Dickens's *A Christmas Carol* revolves around Scrooge's learning that selfishness has destroyed his own life and harmed those around him, and that kindness and mercy offer him hope not only of a spiritual redemption but of a more pleasant earthly existence as well.

Sometimes only the negative consequences of egocentrism are shown, as in *Romeo and Juliet*, where the selfish bitterness of the Montagues and the Capulets destroys their own children.

Sometimes the focus of a story is on the positive results of unselfishness. In Victor Hugo's classic *Les Miserables*, a single act of kindness is shown to a man who had not seen much kindness. His repeated imitation of that act in showing kindness to others results in untold good, like ripples in a pond spreading out from a single pebble.

In the Frank Capra classic film *It's a Wonderful Life*, George Bailey repeatedly gives up his dreams in deference to the welfare of others. He does not see what good his sacrifices have done until he is enlightened through the course of the film. In the end, he sees the gratefulness of the many people he has helped, and he understands that he has gained something more valuable than the world travel and adventures he had wanted.

I would argue that most great works of literature involve a character's growing from egocentrism to a greater understanding of others. Why is awareness of the needs of others such an important theme in literature? Why does self-sacrifice continue to inspire us, even if our own life is focused on ourselves?

Deep down, I believe we all *know* that self-actualization is not our true purpose. I believe that God has put into each of us a desire to reach beyond ourselves and to sacrifice for a greater good. As a Christian, I believe that greater good is in obeying God wherever he leads me, following the example of Jesus, who gave his life for us.

If we have a purpose higher than finding happiness for ourselves, then our physical health may *not* be the most important thing. Hanging onto life is less important than "getting a life," as the saying goes. After we have decided what we believe and why, we need to organize our life around our priorities and accomplish what we believe is important.

We should certainly do everything we can to stay healthy and to take care of ourselves when we face disease. But we should also decide what aspects of our life are more important to us than our physical health.

As noted earlier, it is a frequent observation among doctors that cancer patients are among the nicest people we meet. They focus on those around them and do acts of kindness to help others. In the process, they make their own lives better as well. They do not worry about minor annoyances that are really un-

A Christian Perspective

Spiritual health is more important than physical health. Paul's advice to Timothy in 1 Timothy 4:8 captures this idea perfectly when he says, "For bodily discipline is only of little profit, but godliness is profitable for all things, since it holds promise for the present life and also for the life to come."

important; instead they focus on the things that are truly important.

We would be wise to follow their example. When we face death, we will not measure our life by the length of time we have lived. We will not spend our last hours totaling up the things we have accumulated. We will not just reminisce about the pleasure we have experienced. Instead, we will critically quantify the character we have shown in our actions. We will count up the contributions we have made to the causes that reflect our true, heartfelt beliefs. Most of all, we will ask ourselves how we have cared for those we love.

Conclusion

"Dr. Brown, I have enjoyed talking about these things. You have reminded me that other parts of my life are important. I plan to focus on my children and my husband and to enjoy each day that I have to the fullest. I have been so frightened since the heart attack that I hadn't been able to think of much else."

"Julie, I hope that we can keep you healthy. Let's work on using the best medicines that are available to make your heart strong. Let's avoid medicines that are not likely to help. Let's build good habits and avoid bad ones. But let's always keep our lives in balance, focusing on those things that are most important."

Notes

1. American Cancer Society, "Guidelines for the Early Detection of Cancer," www.cancer.org/docroot/PED/content/PED_2_3X_ACS_Cancer_Detection_Guide lines_36.asp?sitearea=PED (accessed June 19, 2006).

2. C. S. Lewis, *Mere Christianity* (New York: Macmillan, 1971).